Better But Not Well

Better But Not Well

Mental Health Policy in the United States since 1950

RICHARD G. FRANK
AND
SHERRY A. GLIED

Foreword by Rosalynn Carter

The Johns Hopkins University Press
Baltimore

This book was brought to publication with the generous assistance of the
MacArthur Foundation Network on Mental Health Policy Research.

The Johns Hopkins University Press
2715 North Charles Street
Baltimore, Maryland 21218-4363
www.press.jhu.edu

Library of Congress Cataloging-in-Publication Data

Frank, Richard G.
Better but not well : mental health policy in the United States since 1950 / Richard G.
Frank and Sherry A. Glied.
p. ; cm.
Includes bibliographical references and index.
ISBN 0-8018-8442-X (hardcover : alk. paper)—ISBN 0-8018-8443-8 (pbk. : alk. paper)
1. Mental health policy—United States—History. 2. Mental health services—United
States—History.
[DNLM: 1. Mental Health Services—trends—United States—Statistics. 2. Health Policy—
trends—United States—Statistics. 3. Mental Health Services—statistics & numerical data
—United States. WM 30 F828b 2006] I. Glied, Sherry. II. Title.
RA790.6.F723 2006
362.2'0973—dc22
2006001810

A catalog record for this book is available from the British Library.

To our spouses

CONTENTS

America has always struggled to care for and support people who have mental illnesses. The challenges of addressing these disabling health conditions demand that we both show our compassion and use our ingenuity. When Jimmy was president during the 1970s, I served as honorary chairperson for a presidential commission to assess the mental heath needs of the nation and to develop recommendations for meeting these needs. The result of that commission was the enactment of the Mental Health Systems Act of 1980. Unfortunately, the legislation was never funded by the next administration, although much of it was eventually implemented in practice. Twenty-five years later, President George W. Bush established the President's New Freedom Commission on Mental Health. Regrettably, many of the problems noted in the 1970s remain, but there have been some exciting developments, especially the expectation of recovery now for people with mental illnesses.

In considering how to better address the mental health needs of the American people, we must, from time to time, take stock of our successes and failures. In *Better But Not Well,* Professors Frank and Glied offer a broad-based and candid assessment of the evolution of mental health care in the United States and of how the well-being of people touched by mental health problems changed during the last half of the twentieth century. They highlight significant gains in our investments in mental health care, in scientific advances, and in new opportunities for people with mental illnesses to share in everyday life. Frank and Glied also offer a sober examination of some notable failures, including the inexcusable increases in homelessness and incarceration of people who have mental illnesses. Their analysis provides a new understanding of how economic, scientific, and legal forces combined to shape the way people with these disorders are cared for today. Fortunately, they use their assessment to define some new directions for mental health policy in the twenty-first century.

This kind of periodic examination of where mental health care in the United States stands is necessary because so much work remains to be done. For too long, mental illnesses have been shrouded in secrecy, shame, and hopelessness. We must continue to work toward eliminating the stigma surrounding them, abolishing barriers that exclude people with these illnesses from sharing in the benefits of American society, expanding scientific inquiry, and developing policies that serve to promote mental health and prevent mental illnesses. It is my goal to see mental illnesses attended to like all other diseases so that people with them can share fully in everyday life.

Rosalynn Carter
Chair
The Carter Center Mental Health Task Force

In the past ten years, discussions of mental health policy have routinely taken a dour view of the recent history of mental health care in the United States. President Bush's 2003 New Freedom Commission report begins by calling mental health care in America "a system that had fallen into a state of disarray." The Bazelon Center for Mental Health Law's 2001 call to action argues that "for decades mental health systems have been burdened with ineffective service delivery programs and stagnant state bureaucracies" (Bazelon Center, 2001). These views of the past sometimes generate policy proposals that treat existing policies and institutions simply as hopeless impediments to progress. At other times, advocates cling to familiar institutions that have long served people with mental illnesses as "ports in a storm." Yet if their views of the past are distorted, policy makers and advocates may be mistaken in the institutions and policies they choose in an effort to make a better future.

In 1999 the MacArthur Foundation's Network on Mental Health Policy began a series of discussions about how to improve the care of people with mental illness in the United States. It quickly became clear that the discussions were heavily influenced by perceptions of the recent past. We realized that we needed an empirical scorecard that assessed how the well-being of people with mental illness had changed since the policy ferment of the late 1950s and 1960s and what forces had caused the evolution of care. Thus, the Network encouraged us to engage in a data-driven assessment of the recent history of mental health care, and we recognized that we would view the evidence and the events in the delivery of mental health care through the lens of the discipline of economics.

This book is the result of that reexamination. Our purpose is to explore the changes occurring over the last fifty years in the lives of people with mental illnesses and to assess the factors that generated these changes. Discerning if people with mental illnesses are better off turns out to be far from simple. This book strives to collect and analyze the indicators that may be useful to glean a fair and accurate picture of how lives have improved and then to infer why. Emphasizing only the deficiencies of the present—without an understanding of how these relate to the past—can lead to a replay of earlier unproductive efforts. By taking a longer-term view of the subject, we aim to put some of today's problems into perspective. Understanding the forces that have promoted and impeded gains in the lives of people with mental illness can help to guide the development of policies likely to prove useful in the future. This book places special emphasis on how increasing decentralization and declining mental health exceptionalism have contributed to these changes in well-being. Chapter 1 provides an overview of the major developments affecting the well-being of people with mental illness since 1950. In chapter 2 we evaluate estimates of the size and character of the population with mental illness over time. Our analysis suggests that the size of the population with mental illness—or with severe mental illness—has remained relatively constant as a share of the U.S. population. Furthermore, the characteristics of the population with mental illness have not changed substantially over time. Together, these two findings imply that whatever improvement or deterioration we observe in the condition of people with mental illness cannot be attributed mainly to changes in the underlying population.

Chapter 3 turns to a second possible explanation of changes in the well-being of the population with mental illness—changes in the ability to treat illness effectively. The early part of this fifty-year period—the 1950s and 1960s—saw the development of several therapies for the treatment of mental illness that were clearly improvements over the treatments preceding them. Since then, there has been a great deal of innovation. In terms of symptom reduction alone, however, the treatment arsenal available today is not really much better than that available twenty-five years ago. The new technologies are, however, much easier to use in practice. We argue that practice-simplifying innovations of this kind are particularly important in an era of decentralized practice. We also document the treatment improvements that have come about through the withdrawal from practice of ineffective and harmful treatments. Finally, we note that although there has been considerable innovation in developing new types of psychotherapy, there has been much less success in disseminating them. Our results in chapter 3 suggest that improvements in the efficacy of treatment are not the main driver of improvements in well-being.

In chapter 4 we examine how the financing of mental health services changed over time. The introduction of public health and disability insurance programs—particularly Medicaid and Supplemental Security Income—has had three enormous consequences for people with mental illness. First, these programs have vastly expanded the amount of money spent on people with these illnesses, even relative to overall health spending. Second, the programs moved money from traditional mental health institutions into a much more decentralized web of providers. Finally, because the funds flowing to these programs have dramatically exceeded those available to traditional mental health agencies, these programs have in effect wrested control of mental health services away from these traditional bureaucracies. Financing changes have been the main drivers of both the rise of decentralization and the decline of exceptionalism—and hence, we argue, of improvements in well-being.

Contemporaneous with these financing changes has been a significant increase in the supply of mental health providers—both institutions and professionals. We examine these changes in supply in chapter 5 and document enormous increases in both the number and range of service providers. Competition in the supply of psychotherapy and inpatient psychiatric care, in conjunction with managed behavioral health care arrangements that have altered the method of purchasing mental health services, has resulted in lower prices for many mental health services. The result is that one of the central reasons in the past for not fully integrating mental health care into health insurance benefits—cost control—was resolved during the 1990s.

Chapter 6 evaluates the consequences of these financing and supply changes for mental health care policy. We argue that the decline of mental health exceptionalism has left a void in terms of who has responsibility for the population with mental illness. No single agency within each state is responsible. This is particularly problematic for those with severe mental illness who rely on a wide range of largely uncoordinated public programs. While efforts to coordinate services for some may be successful, further improvement in the well-being of people with mental illness depends on developing an understanding of and appreciation for the value of exceptionalism policies across a range of settings and programs outside the mental health field.

In chapter 7 we assess the conditions of people with mental illness. We examine how the population has fared with respect to treatment receipt, the quality of that treatment, financial burden, and living conditions. We conclude that there has been substantial progress in the first three of these outcomes. In terms of living conditions, the picture is somewhat murkier. For most people with severe mental illness, living conditions have improved over time. Most live in the community and have entitlements to a range of public benefits. Yet a small but growing minority of people with severe illness are worse off because they are either homeless or incarcerated. Those who do live in the community and receive public benefits are arguably better off, but their entitlements are meager and leave them with income generally below the federal poverty line. Better off is far from good enough.

Looking forward, we are generally optimistic that progress will continue. There are, however, important lessons to be learned from the experience of the last fifty years that can inform public policy. Our conclusions in chapter 8 focus on these lessons and their implications.

The integration of policies for people with severe mental illnesses into larger programs that address illness, poverty, and disability leaves intact the concerns that originally generated mental health exceptionalism. Thus, while notions of parity and equality have dominated policy debates around insurance coverage for mental health care, strict parity in the administration of social insurance (e.g., public disability and welfare), criminal justice policy, and employment supports may serve to disadvantage people with mental disorders because of their unique needs. Mental health policy has, in effect, moved out of the single state agencies that formerly had responsibility for mental health care; now it must become an explicit concern of the mainstream institutions that oversee public health and social insurance programs, as well as private health care systems. We propose the creation of a new federal agency or authority, reporting to the president, with budgetary oversight of all programs that serve people with mental illness. The purpose of this agency would be to provide a voice for mental health exceptionalism in the context of mainstream programs.

People with mental disorders are among the most vulnerable and disadvantaged members of U.S. society. America's struggle to address mental illness in its population humanely, efficiently, and fairly has advanced greatly. People with mental illness are much better off than they were just fifty years ago. Nevertheless, we remain limited in our ability to reduce many of the disabling and destructive consequences of mental disorders and we frequently fail to provide circumstances that allow people with mental disorders to live with dignity and meet their basic needs. Our system of care is not yet well.

This book has its origins in the John D. and Catherine T. MacArthur Foundation's Network on Mental Health Policy. The network and the foundation provided financial support for the project, and members of the network offered an unending source of expert advice and encouragement. Laurie Garduque of the MacArthur Foundation was unwavering in her encouragement, as was the director of the network, Howard Goldman. Additional financial support was provided by the Center for Mental Health Services in the U.S. Department of Health and Human Services. Bernie Arons and Judith Katz-Levy made that support possible and gave us much guidance.

In undertaking a project that is as broad in scope as this one, we regularly relied on the expertise and assistance of colleagues from other disciplines. We gratefully acknowledge the assistance of Shana McCormack and Adam Neufeld and advice from Audrey Burnam in our work on chapter 2. In writing chapter 3, we relied on clinical and scientific assistance in organizing material and evidence from Alisa Busch, Miriam Davis, Howard Goldman, and Sharon Kofman. Rena Conti provided expert research assistance for chapter 4. Kathrine Jack and Douglas Gould lent programming and research support to chapter 5. Chapters 6 and 7 benefited from assistance from Julie Donohue, Kristina Hanson, and James O'Malley. David Brick, Rachel Clement, and Sarah Little provided research assistance for chapter 7.

Several members of the network devoted a great deal of effort to helping us address difficult issues, including the evolution of mental health law, disparities, children's mental health, and the evolution of the managed behavioral health care industry. We offer special thanks to Saul Feldman, Pam Hyde, Kelly Kelleher, Jeanne Miranda, and Hank Steadman. Several people read and discussed drafts of sections of the book and offered many constructive comments. For this we thank Leon Eisenberg, Tom McGuire, Dan O'Flaherty, Bob Rose, and Diane Rowland. Kris Bolt provided terrific support in the production of the manuscript and the construction of the bibliography.

Better But Not Well

CHAPTER I

Introduction

The mental health system today bears scant resemblance to that of the first half of the twentieth century. Albert Deutsch, after a decade of investigation, indicted mental health care in 1948 in *The Shame of the States*. Deutsch described how people with severe mental illness languished on the filthy back wards of public mental hospitals, lacking any care or being subjected to generally ineffective and often painful therapies. In one provocative passage he wrote of mental hospitals as "buildings swarming with naked humans herded like cattle . . . pervaded by a fetid odor so heavy, so nauseating, that the stench seemed to have almost a physical existence of its own."

For people with mental illness, life outside public mental hospitals was only marginally better. Many of the severely ill eked out an existence, living in squalid hotels or slum apartments with no reliable source of income and little prospect of treatment. Those with less severe illnesses—depression, or anxiety, or phobias— might turn to a sympathetic member of the clergy or a friend, but they had little other recourse. Their physicians' therapeutic arsenal contained only addictive or ineffective medications. Prosperous patients, the privileged few, were likely to receive humane, caring treatment in private psychiatric hospitals or from psychiatrists in private practice. But the treatment itself was not much more effective than that received by their more disadvantaged peers.

Over the second half century, from 1950 to 2000, there occurred a dramatic transformation in the way the United States addressed the needs of people with mental illnesses. Today the vast majority— even those with a severe illness— never see the inside of a public mental hospital. Almost all severely ill patients receive some treatment. That treatment, although not always entirely effective, is unlikely to be dangerous or inhumane. The living conditions of people with severe illnesses have generally improved at least as much as have conditions for the rest of society over the past five decades.

Most severely ill people today receive regular income through federal insurance programs, and their medical care, in the community and in hospitals, is paid for by public or private insurance. A small army of specialty-trained psychiatrists, psychologists, nurses, and social workers, who collectively number more than two hundred thousand, has replaced the seven thousand psychiatrists practicing in 1950. Family doctors who had long ignored mental health problems now assume an active role in the management of many psychiatric illnesses. Average spending on care for each person treated has expanded many times over, even after accounting for inflation. People with mental illnesses, their families, and the population at large have better financial protection against the costs of mental illness. And people with mental illness share more civil liberties. The courts have restored their dignity by extending new rights protecting them from being hospitalized against their will. Many now lead productive lives as active members of their communities. The result is that the lives of most people with mental illnesses are better today than they were fifty years ago.

Undoubtedly, the circumstances of people with mental illness remain far from acceptable. President Bush's New Freedom Commission of 2003 reported that the mental health system is "in shambles." The report described excessive disability, homelessness, dependence on social programs, school failure, and incarceration in jails and prisons. Though evidence of improvement is abundant, the picture we sketch should not obscure how extraordinarily disruptive mental illnesses remain. People with severe mental disorders still have among the lowest rates of employment of any group with disabilities. Their earnings are lower and they are less likely to return to work than are other people with disabilities. The World Health Organization calculated that mental illnesses lead to a greater collective disability burden in established market economies than does any other group of illnesses, including cancer and heart disease (WHO, 2001).

Mentally ill people disproportionately populate the nation's largest social insurance programs. They account for up to 35 percent of those on public disability and 28 percent on welfare rolls (Loprest and Zedlewski, 1999; US SSA, 2001). As we will show, the growth of these mainstream social insurance programs has been vitally important in improving the circumstances of people with mental illness. Nonetheless, public disability insurance does not pay enough to lift an adult above the federal poverty line. For the vast majority of people with a severe mental illness, a life in poverty is to be expected; it is almost preordained from the moment of diagnosis, which is often by late adolescence.

Mental illness may lead to homelessness or incarceration, often both. An estimated 30 percent of homeless single adults have a serious mental illness, as do a disproportionate share of those in jails and prisons (Teplin, 1990; Burt, 2001). The public, in the abstract, is more optimistic about treating mental illnesses. But on a personal level members of the public still wish to keep their distance. People with mental illnesses may lose many of their civil rights and their liberty, either through civil commitment or by being arrested for minor crimes arising from their erratic behavior. Even people with less severe mental illnesses can experience significant income loss, family disruption, drug abuse, and stigmatization. People with severe mental illnesses remain among the most gravely disadvantaged and stigmatized groups in the United States.

The report of the U.S. surgeon general of 1999 detailed the rich array of effective treatments for mental illnesses that existed by the end of the twentieth century, but it also pointed out that many people never receive these treatments and that the quality of treatment is highly uneven. Some 40 percent of people with private insurance receive treatments for major depression that are completely ineffective (Berndt et al., 2002). Only half the people treated for schizophrenia receive evidence-based care (Lehman and Steinwachs, 1998).

Though most people today have public or private health insurance to cover the costs of mental health care, the financial burden of treating these illnesses can still be crushing. Health insurance plans commonly impose special limits on coverage for mental illness. The limits usually are on the number of days of hospitalization or of outpatient visits. In fact, limits of this sort turn the concept of true insurance on its head: the most valuable part of insurance is that which protects against the catastrophic costs of an illness. This coverage may leave someone to face financial ruin in the event of serious illness.

Thus, although there have been substantial improvements in the care and support of mentally ill people, their situation today is far from ideal. The current state of people with mental illness echoes the conclusion made more than twenty-five years ago by the psychiatrist Gerald Klerman. As the director of federal research and service programs, he characterized individuals with mental illnesses as "better but not well" (Klerman, 1977).

Why Has Well-being Improved?

The well-being of people with mental illness has been the subject of copious scholarly study, multiple distinguished committees, costly demonstration projects, public relations campaigns, and billions of dollars of scientific research. One of our recurrent findings is that improvements in the condition of people with mental illness have come about largely irrespective of these focused efforts. Nor do improvements stem primarily from monumental scientific breakthroughs in the efficacy of treatment (at least since the 1960s).

Rather, these improvements have evolved through avenues that in other contexts would seem obvious: more money, greater consumer choice, and the increased competition among technologies and providers that these forces unleashed. The passage of Medicaid and Medicare in the mid-1960s was a boon to people with high health care needs, including those with mental illness. The new federal funding led to a gradual and steady adaptation of existing mental health care systems. This process moved resources out of the existing networks of bureaucracies, hospitals, and professionals and into new agencies and provider groups. Expansions in the scope and generosity of private insurance that continued through the 1990s had the same effect in the private sector. The introduction in 1972 of Supplemental Security Income (SSI) disability benefits for the first time furnished direct income to many with severe mental illnesses, which improved both their absolute and relative well-being. Health insurance and disability benefits put money and choices into the hands of people with mental illness, rather than into the hands of their service providers and caretakers. Consumerism and markets transformed the mental health system.

A similar process led to greater civil rights for people with mental illness. Buoyed by their successes in the civil rights movement, many advocates of civil liberties turned their attention toward other disenfranchised groups, including people with mental illness. Several landmark court decisions mandated that people with mental illness be given the right to participate actively in treatment and commitment decisions, and that restrictions on their freedom could not be imposed casually. These decisions further encouraged patient autonomy and consumerism. They also led to increases in the costs of public mental hospitals, which created more impetus for community-based treatment. Later the Americans with Disabilities Act of 1990 incorporated mental illness into its broad sweep; it held that employers had to make reasonable accommodations that might permit people with mental illness to work. These legal requirements enabled people to make choices about how to live their lives and to participate in decisions about their treatment.

Funding growth and regulatory changes promoted the entry into the market of new groups of professionals. Unprecedented increases in the number of mental health professionals, which persisted into the 1990s, flooded the market with treatment options. The supply of physicians also increased greatly over this period, and primary care physicians and pediatricians became more interested in treating mental health conditions. The number of private psychiatric hospital beds also grew rapidly beginning in the 1980s.

Funding growth and regulatory change also had seismic effects on the public mental health system, which, from its origins in the nineteenth century, was based on centralized state mental health organizations. Funds from each state legislature flowed to a specialized set of institutions and providers, usually through the state's mental health authority or mental health agency. Today, by contrast, the system has become decentralized, so much so that the term *system* borders on a misnomer. Individuals with a mental illness have flexible entitlements to an array of largely uncoordinated programs and resources, including medical care and income support. The resources flow from a dizzying range of federal, state, and private organizations. One estimate of programs at the federal level alone sets the total at more than forty (Parrott and Dean, 2002).

Mental health services—for those with severe or not so severe illness—are no longer as distinctive, with their own set of dedicated providers, institutions, and policy-making bodies. Today people with severe mental illness receive benefits largely from programs that also serve people with other disabling conditions. People with mental illnesses of all types have their medical care paid for by the same organizations that pay for physical health care. Mental health care has been mainstreamed.

Finally, the expanded financial and professional resources available for treating people with mental illness and the legally and culturally instigated focus on patient participation in treatment made possible a lucrative new market for all sorts of therapies. This market depended not only on the effectiveness of these therapies, but also on the abilities of patients to comply with prescription instructions and of practitioners to prescribe new therapies appropriately. Entrepreneurs at pharmaceutical firms, providers, and hospitals responded to these new market incentives by generating options that would attract patients. These treatments often do not produce notably higher rates of symptom alleviation in clinical trials. Instead, they are popular because they are safer, easier to tolerate, and easier to prescribe than were their predecessors.

Taken together, new treatment options such as selective serotonin reuptake inhibitor pharmaceutical agents (SSRIs such as Prozac and Zoloft), new providers of psychotherapy (social workers and counselors), and a range of private psychiatric inpatient providers (for-profit and nonprofit) have been extraordinarily financially successful. Their success, in turn, spurred efforts by payers to ration care more strictly. These efforts, culminating (so far) in the emergence of managed behavioral health care plans that today dominate mental health financing, further reconfigured the mental health system. This system attempts—at least in its rhetoric—to allocate care according to the costs and documented effectiveness of therapies, in the context of considerable consumer choice.

Mental Health Exceptionalism: Past and Future

In some respects, mental illness poses unique public policy problems. Unlike many other disabling conditions, mental illness can, by its nature, impede people's abilities to make decisions about their own care. People with mental illness also pose unique challenges to society. Mental illness can disrupt communities and, in some situations, is associated with a heightened risk of violent behavior.

At the same time, many of the other problems that complicate mental health policy making are not unique to mental health care. Variations in the quality and use of services have been documented throughout medical care. Containing the costs of care is a challenge throughout the health care system. Private insurance markets suffer from a variety of incentive and information problems; of these, adverse selection—when people choose to purchase insurance coverage (or choose which type of coverage to purchase) on the basis of their own information about their likely need for services—is among the most mischievous. The design of social insurance is also complex. The U.S. social safety net has many holes. These problems, though, are magnified in the context of mental illness.

In keeping with the severity and unique features of policy problems in mental health, for most of the past century mental illness has been addressed very differently from other health problems. It has partly been viewed like any other set of illnesses needing compassionate care, but it is also seen as a threat to law and order. The treatment of some mental disorders that involved ordinary quirks and complaints was ridiculed as a self-indulgent luxury, even a pretext for avoiding adult responsibilities. Conversely, treatment for schizophrenia and other severe disorders was considered so essential to protecting self and others that society felt justified in forcing people to be medicated against their will.

The distinctiveness of mental health policy problems led to the development of an institutional structure centered around specialty mental health systems run primarily by state mental health agencies (SMHA). The SMHA provided a guaranteed supply of specialized care, political focus for advocates, and state police powers for social control. The policies that guided these centralized state systems were prime examples of what we call mental health *exceptionalism*. We define exceptionalism as policies that exclusively focus on mental illness.

Since the 1960s, however, policies of exceptionalism have been on the decline. Mental health advocates have sought integration into the mainstream of health care. They have actively supported an end to discrimination against mental illness, especially in health insurance. They have aggressively advocated for more biomedical research funding and welcomed the march of science and a biomedical orientation to illness. In short, they have pursued policies placing mental illness on an even footing with other health care concerns. They have demanded that policy makers cease segregating mental health and incorporate it fully into general health policy. Their triumph was on prominent display in 1999, when Surgeon General David Satcher declared in his preface to the first-ever surgeon general's report on mental health: "Leaders in the mental health field—fiercely dedicated advocates, scientists, government officials, and consumers—have been insistent that mental health flow in the mainstream of health. I agree and issue this report in that spirit" (US DHHS, CMHS, 1999).

But integration into the mainstream has significant disadvantages. Exceptionalism offered the opportunity for policy makers to provide distinctive—arguably preferential—options for people with mental illness. The state mental health systems' ability to influence mental health policy and offer such distinctive benefits has now been vastly curtailed. Further, many of the key forces that prompted policies of exceptionalism are still in place, including stigma, discrimination, inequities, adverse selection, and the need for social control. The special challenges have not diminished. The state bureaucracies that were charged with guaranteeing access to mental health care and ensuring the quality of services have been weakened. The policy makers with the greatest clout over mental health care today sit in offices scattered over every level of government—Medicaid agencies, state welfare departments, the Social Security Administration, and the Department of Corrections. Institutions and professions that specialize in the treatment of mental illness have had to accept a diminished role in the delivery of care. Efforts to unite these programs under a mental health agency umbrella have not been successful in improving outcomes of care.

CHAPTER 2

The Population with Mental Illness

Mental illness is far more visible today than it was fifty years ago. People with severe mental illness, once housed in state institutions often located far from population centers, now live in the community. People who were once thought to have personality quirks or to be victims of harsh social circumstances are now described in medical terms as having symptoms of a disorder. Many newspapers now feature stories about mental illness as prominently as stories about cancer. Over this same period there have been radical changes in U.S. society. The divorce rate has tripled. The rate of single parenthood has more than tripled (from about 4% to about 13%). Many more women work in the formal labor market. Men's jobs have become more unstable. These and many other transformations in society and the economy might have triggered an increase in mental illness. Do the growing awareness and visibility of mental illness or the increased stresses of today's world mean that its prevalence over the past five decades has been rising? Rising prevalence of mental illness—if true—would confound our analysis of the last half century of changes in the well-being of people with mental illness. If mental illness has grown in prevalence or strikes different groups from those it once did, then these shifting population patterns may be responsible for the historical changes in well-being.

What Is Mental Illness?

How mental illness is defined over time has been the focus of philosophical debates about the nature of rationality, sociological debates about the meaning of deviance, and legal debates about the definition of criminal responsibility. Advances in social attitudes, scientific understanding, treatment modalities, and diagnostic technology alter the definition of many illnesses over time (Rosenberg, 2002).[1] The problems of defining who has an illness and who does not are far more difficult in the case of mental illness than in the case of most somatic illnesses, however, because few mental disorders have biological markers.

Experts continue to spar about the inclusion of specific conditions in each update of the psychiatric diagnosis manual *Diagnostic and Statistical Manual of Mental Disorders,* the latest of which, published in 2000, is known as DSM-IV-TR (APA, 2000). Even after conditions are identified, epidemiologists argue about how best to measure them in the general population. The balance in these ongoing debates has shifted over time. In earlier eras pitched battles occurred between those favoring more theoretical and personality-oriented categories and those endorsing more medical categories that use a list of signs and symptoms. Recent scientific research has shown how particular mental illnesses cluster in families, how they display similar symptom profiles across diverse cultures and communities, how they follow a predictable course and natural history, and how they respond to treatment (Robins and Guze, 1970; US DHHS, CMHS, 1999). The disabling nature of mental illnesses, especially schizophrenia, major depression, and bipolar disorder, is now abundantly clear (WHO, 2001). Today a medical approach to mental illness is standard.

Epidemiologists have used three general sets of constructs (and combinations of these) to define who has a mental illness. One set focuses on symptoms and signs for each particular mental disorder. A second assesses whether a person has mental health-related difficulties in functioning at school, at work, or at home. A third measures whether a person has sought treatment for a mental health condition.

The differences among these constructs reflect, in part, the diversity of conditions grouped in the umbrella category of mental illness. Some people are universally acknowledged to be very ill, so impaired in their functioning that state law often requires them to be hospitalized whether or not they want treatment. This small group of severely and persistently mentally ill people accounts for most of the costs of mental health care.

A larger group has symptoms that are not as outwardly bizarre or debilitating but that seriously impede their ability to live happy, productive lives. Many with major depression and severe anxiety disorders fall into this category.

Others experience an impaired ability to live their lives because of external events, such as the death of a family member. They may benefit from counseling or treatment but often do not meet criteria for a psychiatric diagnosis. Still others have symptoms consistent with a mental disorder, but the symptoms rarely affect their daily lives.

Finally, a relatively small group believes that therapy is useful as a road to self-discovery. Members of this group and the therapists who treat them would agree that they are not being treated for a mental illness. Although people in this group do not account for a large fraction of current spending on care, they are important for the design of mental health policy because their use of mental health services is highly responsive to price. Generous insurance coverage, which reduces the price of care, can dramatically increase their use of services.

Assessments of the size and composition of the population with mental illness have, at various times, included different combinations of these groups. There is no reason to expect that the different constructs of mental illness—whether by symptoms and signs, functional impairment, or treatment use—will yield the same or similar-sized populations. As the examples above suggest, some people in treatment neither are functionally disabled nor exhibit characteristic symptoms. But many who are functionally disabled or experience characteristic symptoms are not in treatment. People with functional disability may not exhibit symptoms for any one particular disorder, or they may have difficulty functioning because of particular adverse events, such as loss of a loved one, that explain any symptoms.[2]

Each construct selects a distinct subgroup of the population who experience mental health problems, so assessments based on different constructs can generate different estimates of the number of people with mental illness. We examined the overlap between estimates based on these divergent constructs using one of the most recent epidemiologic surveys, the National Comorbidity Survey (NCS). The NCS, conducted between 1990 and 1992 and covering the U.S. noninstitutionalized adult population between ages fifteen and fifty-four, contains good measures of all three constructs: symptom-, treatment-, and impairment-based criteria (NCS described in Kessler et al., 1994). Figure 2.1 shows the overlaps between the percentages meeting criteria for treatment, symptom constellations, and functional disability.

As Figure 2.1 shows, the overlap between the populations described by each of the three constructs is quite small. Less than 2 percent of the entire U.S. adult population falls into all three groups. More than two-thirds of those meeting symptom criteria neither experienced functional disability nor received treatment. One-fourth with a functional disability did not meet symptom criteria. One-fourth in treatment did not report functional impairment and did not meet symptom criteria. Each way that mental illness was defined and measured led to a different prevalence rate: nearly 30 percent using diagnosis and less than 10 percent using either treatment or impairment criteria.

Epidemiologists generally prefer the use of a combination of criteria to define the population with mental illness. Nonetheless, the most widely cited estimates of the prevalence of mental illness, drawn from the NCS and from the Epidemiologic Catchment Area study (of adults), provide a one-year prevalence of a diagnosable

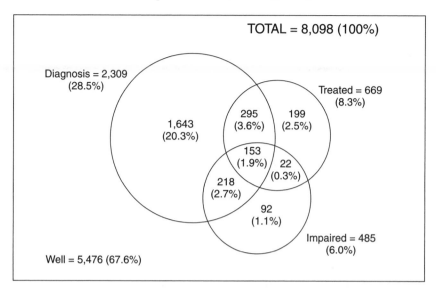

Figure 2.1. National Comorbidity Survey (1994), Venn Diagram. The figures for Diagnosis, Impaired, and Treated include overlap.
SOURCE: Data from Kessler et al., 1994.

mental disorder based on symptoms alone in 28–30 percent of adults (one-year prevalence refers to the percentage of the population meeting criteria for a diagnosable illness over a twelve-month period). The addition of impairment criteria substantially reduces the estimated prevalence of mental illness to about 20–22.5 percent (Bird et al., 1990; Narrow et al., 2002; Regier and Narrow, 2002).[3]

The definition of mental illness reflected in this prevalence estimate remains quite broad. Many people within this category have illnesses that may be relatively mild or transient. Just as a substantial proportion of the population meets diagnostic criteria and experiences some impairment from a physical condition, a substantial proportion experiences a diagnosable mental illness. As we describe below, only a small subgroup of this population has a serious and persistent mental illness.

Sociodemographic Characteristics of People with Mental Illness

We analyzed epidemiologic studies conducted over the past fifty years (table 2.1) to assess whether the composition of the population with mental illness has been changing. The earliest study was published in 1944, and the most recent in 2005. Our focus is on adults, because only a handful of studies over this period focused on children, and those few covered small geographical areas, not nation-

TABLE 2.1
Studies That Estimate the Size of the Population with Mental Illness

Study (year)	No. of Subjects	Diagnostic Criteria
Boston Area Induction Station Sel. Service (1942) (Hyde and Kingsley, 1944)	60,000	Mobilization regulations (1942)
Army (1942–45) (U.S. Army Medical Service, 1966)	41,837,088	Mobilization regulations (1942)
Hutterite communities (1950) (Eaton and Weil, 1955)	8,542	DSM-I (APA, 1952)
Salt Lake City, Utah (1955) (Cole et al., 1957)	175 HH	Symptomatology, hospital admission
Baltimore noninstitutional (1957) (Commission on Chronic Illness, 1957)	809	DSM-I (APA, 1952)
Baltimore community (1957) (Pasamanick et al., 1959)[a]	12,000	DSM-I (APA, 1952) severity of impairment
New Haven, Conn. (1958) (Hollingshead and Redlich, 1958)[b]	238,831	In-patient status
Hunterdon County, N.J. (1959) (Trussell et al., 1956)	13,113	AMA, WHO classifications
Midtown Manhattan (1962) (Srole, 1962)[a]	1,660	Mental health ratings
"Stirling County" (1963) (Leighton et al., 1963)[a]	1,010	DSM-I (APA, 1952)
Washington Heights, N.Y. (1971) (Dohwenrend et al., 1971)	257	Symptomatology, psych. interview
Alachua County, Fla. (1972) (Schwab and Warheit, 1972)	1,645	Symptomatology, self-report
Indian village (Pacific northwest) (1973) (Shore et al., 1973)	100	Health and habit records
New Haven, Conn. (1975–76) (Weissman et al., 1978)	511	SADS-RDC (1977)
ECA (1980) (Robins and Regier, 1991)	20,862	DSM-III (APA, 1980)
NCS (1994) (Kessler et al., 1994)	8,098	DSM-III-R
NCS-R (2001–3) (Kessler et al., 2005)	9,282	DSM-IV

NOTE: In some cases, one-month prevalence is assumed to be equivalent to current prevalence.
[a]Households.
[b]Hospital.
[c]Prevalence of psychiatric "impairment" was measured in these studies.
[d]Measures prevalence of any "probable diagnosis."
[e]Schedule for Affective Disorder and Schizophrenia Research Diagnostic Criteria.

ally representative samples (Costello et al., 1996; Shaffer et al., 1996). In the adult studies we examined the correlation between mental illness and age, gender, race, marital status, socioeconomic status, and living in an urban area (urbanness), factors that have been consistently measured over time in most large epidemiologic surveys.[4] Because we compared rates across surveys that often used different metrics, we reported relative rates of prevalence within the same survey (e.g., the rate of prevalence of one group within the survey relative to another).

Age

Comparing across studies conducted over fifty years, we found that most symptom-based studies show an inverted U-shaped pattern in prevalence across age groups (fig. 2.2). Rates first increase and then decline with age. The peak prevalence is among people in their twenties. Impairment-based studies, by contrast, tend to find an increasing prevalence of psychiatric impairment with age. This pattern suggests that the influence of specific symptoms on the ability to function varies over the life cycle. Older adults with the same sets of symptoms as younger adults find their ability to function more compromised. The overall conclusion we draw is that age and mental illness have had a very stable relationship over these fifty years.

Gender

Most studies, whether based on impairment or symptoms, find relatively similar rates of illness among women and men. Nevertheless, the overall gender ratio in a given study strongly depends on whether it includes or excludes substance use disorders. Substance abuse is, in study after study, found more commonly in men. Depression and other affective disorders, on the other hand, are higher in women (e.g., Kessler et al., 1994). Usually the two offset each other, so the overall rate of mental illness is the same across the sexes.

Race

Many studies in the 1950s and 1960s found higher rates of mental illness among nonwhites (mostly blacks). Researchers interpreted this as demonstrating that pervasive discrimination and other social ills facing minorities caused them to develop mental illness. If this was true, changes in civil rights and in economic opportunities might have had a substantial effect on the sociodemographic composition of mental illness. In practice, however, most epidemiologic studies included very small samples of nonwhites, which limited the ability to make race-specific inferences from them. Two studies conducted thirty-five years apart included large nonwhite samples and failed to find higher rates of mental illness in minorities (Pasamanick et al., 1959, 97; Kessler et al., 1994). By con-

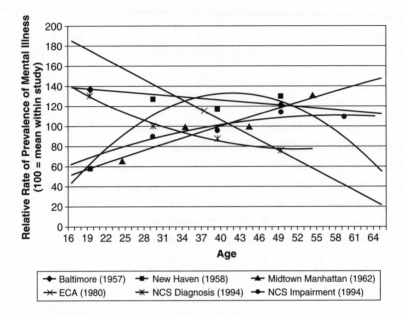

Figure 2.2. Relationship of Age to Relative Risk of Prevalence of Mental Illness in Five Studies, 1957–1994

sources: Data for New Haven (1958) from Hollingshead and Redlich, 1958. Data for Baltimore Community (1957) from Pasamanick, 1959. Data for Midtown Manhattan (1962) from Srole, 1962. Data for ECA (1980) from Robins and Regier, 1991. Data for NCS Diagnosis and NCS Impairment from Kessler et al., 1994.

trast, the 1991 ECA did find a higher overall rate of mental disorders among blacks.[5] Nonetheless, there does not seem to be a systematic trend over time in the relative prevalence of symptoms or impaired functioning by race.

Socioeconomic Status

The strongest and most stable relationship in a half century of studies is between mental illness and socioeconomic status (SES), whether measured using income, education, or occupation. We looked at SES in relation to mental illness across the same studies covering the period from 1950 to 2000. We compared prevalence by SES group, measuring SES as a percentile of the median in that study's population. We used this measure because the definition of SES differed across studies and overall levels of income and education also changed. This relative measure allows us to make consistent comparisons across studies and over time.

The prevalence of mental illness was uniformly highest among the lowest SES

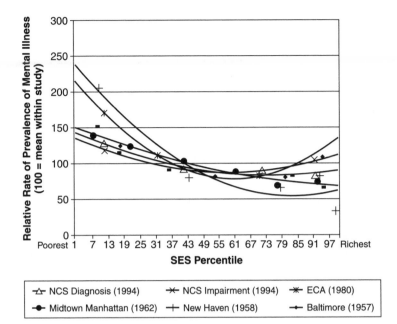

Figure 2.3. Relationship of Socioeconomic Status (SES) to Mental Health Status in Six Studies, 1957–1994

SOURCES: Data for New Haven (1958) from Hollingshead and Redlich, 1958. Data for Baltimore Community (1957) from Pasamanick, 1959. Data for Midtown Manhattan (1962) from Srole, 1962. Data for ECA (1980) from Robins and Regier, 1991. Data for NCS Diagnosis and NCS Impairment from Kessler et al., 1994.

groups. This finding was so strong that it did not vary by how mental illness was defined or measured (fig. 2.3).

A persistent problem in measuring the relationship of SES and mental illness is causality: is mental illness caused by poverty and other social inequalities (social causality) or do people with mental illness become poor because of their illness (reverse causality)? To avoid these problems, many of the surveys we examined measured SES using characteristics less likely to be caused by mental illness, such as parents' income or the individual's education.[6] Our comparison across studies generally suggests that the relationship between SES and mental illness is not—and has not in the past—been *entirely* due to reverse causality. The relationship is roughly the same for those studies that use current income and those studies that use these other measures.

In general, these studies suggest that the relationship between demographic characteristics and mental illness—defined either by the presence of symptoms or by functional impairment—has remained quite stable over time. The prevalence of mental illness is greatest among those in the lowest socioeconomic status groups and varies little by ethnicity or gender. Functional impairment tends to increase with age (among adults), while the prevalence of symptoms is flat (or even declining) in age.

Estimates of Population Size

Estimates of the number of people with mental illness have been made at several points over the past five decades (see table 2.1). The earlier studies varied considerably in their methods and in their rigor. Moreover, until very recently, most surveys have examined the prevalence of mental illness in small and distinct subsamples of the population. The groups are usually defined by residence (one or several counties or cities) and sometimes by other characteristics (army recruits; Amish people). Few of the surveys included people who were incarcerated (Robins and Regier, 1991). The surveys also varied substantially in size—from surveys of just one hundred people in an American Indian village (Shore et al., 1973) to more than 41 million entering the army (U.S. Army Medical Service, 1966). The variability in quality and samples across the studies makes it difficult to discern prevalence trends over time.

Only a few studies—recent or historic—included the inpatient hospital population (Hollingshead and Redlich, 1958). The omission might be important because the fraction of the inpatient population with mental illness is almost certainly very high. Yet even at the height of institutionalization in the mid-1950s, only a tiny fraction of Americans—fewer than 0.5 of 1 percent—were residents of mental hospitals.[7] Similarly, the U.S. prison population today stands at 1.8 million people, of whom an estimated 200,000—less than 1 percent of the U.S. adult population—have a serious mental illness. Exclusion of the institutionalized population could, however, lead to significant underestimates of the population with severe illness because the prevalence of severe illness in the general population is much lower and this group is more likely to be institutionalized.

Studies vary in the construct that the researchers sought to measure (symptoms or impairment or both). Yet even when researchers agree on the underlying construct they wish to measure, changing knowledge about treatment, impairment, or diagnosis leads to shifting definitions of mental illness.[8] As new treatments are introduced, the definition of the population treated expands to incorporate those using these treatments; as old treatments are discarded, the people using them will no longer be counted. Whether someone is functionally impaired depends critically on how functioning is defined. The definition fluctuates over time with ideas about what it means to be productive. For example, if women are not expected to participate in the paid labor force, then a woman's inability to participate would not be considered an impairment.

The definition of what is and what is not a mental disorder also can dramatically affect prevalence rates over time. Scholarly debates hinge on whether behavior departing from social norms is abnormal enough to be labeled a mental illness. Some behaviors previously viewed as disorders, and thus considered abnormal, have been removed from the list, while others have been introduced over time.[9]

Consider the fierce debates surrounding the diagnosis of attention deficit hyperactivity disorder (ADHD), the most commonly diagnosed and treated psychiatric disorder of children. Prevalence rates for ADHD have skyrocketed over the past decade (Robison et al., 1999), but some critics argue that current diagnostic criteria "medicalize" what are otherwise normal variations in child behavior or appropriate responses to disturbing environments (NIH Consensus Statement, 1998).

These definitional changes over time naturally have an effect on the number of people estimated to have a particular disorder and, as a result, the rate of mental illness overall. The results of two large-scale studies conducted less than a decade and a half apart, the National Comorbidity Survey (NCS) and the Epidemiologic Catchment Area study (ECA), seem to vary (substantially for some disorders) because of the differences in diagnostic criteria. The NCS relied on the 1987 criteria of the DSM-III-R (APA, 1987), whereas the ECA relied on the earlier criteria of the DSM-III (APA, 1979). How each anxiety disorder is defined has a noticeable influence. In the most dramatic example, the prevalence of social phobia in the ECA was 2.5 percent, compared to 8.1 percent in the NCS. The seeming rise in the overall rate of anxiety disorders probably reflects shifting diagnostic criteria rather than a true change in prevalence (Regier et al., 1998).

As this discussion suggests, it is difficult to directly compare measures of mental illness from different surveys taken at different times because of varying constructs of mental illness and the instruments used to measure them. Table 2.2 provides the best estimates, from each of the surveys described in table 2.1, of the prevalence of mental illness at each point in time. Table 2.2 conveys the nature and extent of prevalence variations across surveys.

The prevalence of mental illness (six months to one year) ranges between a low of nearly 10 percent and a high of just over 30 percent. This range excludes the New Haven study, which sampled only institutionalized people, and the very small study of a Native American village. There is expected variation, depending on which groups are sampled and which constructs are employed (diagnosis or

TABLE 2.2
The Prevalence of Mental Illness

Study (Year)	Prevalence (%)				
	Lifetime	12-Month	3-Month	Current	Impairment
Boston Area Induction Station Sel. Service (1942) (Hyde and Kingsley, 1944)	—	—	—	10.60	—
Army (1942–45) (U.S. Army Medical Service, 1966)	—	—	—	9.82	—
Hutterite communities (1950) (Eaton and Weil, 1955)	—	—	16.7	0.55	—
Salt Lake City, Utah (1955) (Cole et al., 1957)	—	—	—	33.30	—
Baltimore noninstitutional (1957) (Commission on Chronic Illness, 1957)	—	11.00	—	—	2.0
Baltimore Community (1957) (Pasamanick et al., 1959)	—	—	—	12.83	—
New Haven, Conn. (1958) (Hollingshead and Redlich, 1958)	—	—	—	0.79	—
Hunterdon County, N.J. (1959) (Trussell et al., 1956)	—	—	—	13.80	—
Midtown Manhattan (1962) (Srole, 1962)	—	—	—	—	23.4
"Stirling County" (1963) (Leighton et al., 1963)	57.0	—	—	20.70	24.0
Washington Heights, N.Y. (1971) (Dohwenrend et al., 1971)	—	—	—	21.79	—
Alachua County, Fla. (1972) (Schwab and Warheit, 1972)	—	—	—	31.10	—
Indian village (Pacific Northwest) (1973) (Shore et al., 1973)	—	—	—	69.00	—
New Haven, Conn. (1975–76) (Weissman et al., 1978)	—	—	—	17.80	—
ECA (1980) (Robins and Regier, 1980)	32.0	20.0	—	15.40	—
NCS (1994) (Kessler et al., 1994)	48.0	29.5	—	—	—
NCS-R (2001–3) (Kessler et al., 2005)	—	26.2	—	—	—

functioning). But there are also very substantial differences between surveys using similar populations and similar constructs. For example, studies using DSM-I reported prevalence only about half as high as studies using DSM-III. Early studies using impairment measures (such as the Army Induction and Selective Service studies) found prevalence half as high as those in Midtown Manhattan

TABLE 2.3
Studies That Estimate the Size of the Population with Severe Mental Illness

Study	Survey	No. of Subjects	Diagnostic Criteria	Prevalence (rate)
Ashbaugh et al., 1983	a. 1972 Survey of Disabled and Nondisabled Persons b. Survey of Disability and Work	a. 18,000 (11,700 chronically disabled, 5,100 nondisabled, 1,200 recently disabled) b. 9,859	Chronically mentally ill (CMI): —Disability: limited in ability to work —Duration (incl. expected): 12 mo. —Diagnostic: main cause is mental illness or chronic nervous disorder	1.03 and 1.07 million (20–64-year-old population) (1%)
Barker et al., 1992	National Health Interview Survey—Mental Health Supplement	113,000	Serious mental illness (SMI): Daily life was "seriously interfered with" by a psychiatric disorder in past 12 mo.	2.7 million (18–64-year-old population) (1.8%)
Kessler et al., 1996	a. National Comorbidity Survey b. Baltimore Epidemiologic Catchment Area study Follow-up	a. 8,098 b. ~3,000	Severe and persistent mental illness (SMI): a. DSM-III-R b. DSM-III disorders: schizophrenia and related disorders, manic-depressive (bipolar) disorder, autism and related disorders, as well as severe forms of major depression, panic disorder, and obsessive-compulsive disorder	4.5 million (18+ population) (2.8%; 3.3% for 18–54)
Minkoff, 1978	Urban Institute estimates using census and National Center for Health Statistics data		Severely disabled: —Noninstitutional: unable to work —Institutional: in institution for more than 30 days	1.45 million (18–64-year-old population) (1.2%)

(23.4%). Overall, the prevalence estimates from successive epidemiologic surveys suggest that between 10 and 30 percent of the population each year experience a diagnosable mental illness. There are no discernible patterns over time within this broad range of estimates.

Several of these studies also calculated proportions of the population with specific diagnoses or in specific diagnostic groups. Estimates of the proportion of the sampled population with specific diagnoses vary substantially. Even the prevalence of a severe disorder, schizophrenia, varies by a factor of 5 across studies, from 0.23 percent (defined broadly as all psychoses) in the 1945 Army Induction Study to 0.5 percent (twelve-month prevalence defined as nonaffective psychosis) in the NCS and 1 percent (twelve-month prevalence defined as schizophrenia, and including an inpatient sample) in the ECA.[10] Large differences are also found for illnesses such as depression and neuroses.

Another set of studies has computed the prevalence of serious mental illness by focusing on functioning. These studies are summarized in table 2.3. Ashbaugh et al. (1983) used the 1972 Survey of Disabled and Nondisabled persons and the 1978 Survey of Disability and Work to estimate a prevalence of 1.03 and 1.07 million, respectively, for the population between twenty and sixty-four years old. These amount to a prevalence of 9.8 and 8.96, respectively, per 1,000 population, nearly 1 percent of the population. Using a slightly broader definition of disability, Barker et al. (1992) used the 1989 Supplement to the National Health Interview Survey to estimate a prevalence of 2.7 million in the adult population between eighteen and sixty-four years of age (17.7 per 1,000 population, nearly 2% of the population). In the mid-1970s Kenneth Minkoff used estimates of the national disabled population from the Urban Institute to estimate a prevalence of 1.5 million people in the adult nonelderly population who had a psychiatric disability (Minkoff, 1978).

Kessler and his colleagues (1996) used the DSM-III-R as diagnostic criteria and estimated that 5.4 percent of adults have a "serious mental illness." The results are based on the National Comorbidity Survey and the follow-up Baltimore Epidemiologic Catchment Area study. Using these studies, Kessler and his colleagues also estimated the prevalence of a more intense mental disorder, "severe and persistent mental illness," to be 2.8 percent of all adults.

Alternative Approaches

Our comparison of estimates of mental illness or of severe and persistent mental illness across the existing epidemiologic surveys reveals wide ranges of estimates but no discernible trend over time. We next considered two alternative approaches to the assessment of changes in the prevalence of mental illness over time.

Cross-Cohort Studies

One way to assess changes in prevalence over time is to compare reported lifetime prevalence for different generations, known as birth cohorts, in the same cross-sectional survey. This approach avoids problems of changing constructs and methods. Several studies have applied this cross-cohort method to studying prevalence rates of depression over time.

Many such studies report that depression in more recent generations has a higher lifetime prevalence and an earlier age of onset than in earlier generations (Klerman et al., 1985; Wickramaratne et al., 1989; Cross-National Collaborative Group, 1992). The size of the difference is enormous. Taken together, the studies suggest that lifetime risk of depression among recent generations is about five times higher than that among those born at the beginning of the twentieth century (Simon and VonKorff, 1992).

A potential problem with examining trends in cross-sectional studies is the possibility of recall bias (ibid.). Older generations might not recall their past mental health as well as younger generations do. Consistent with this view is the fact that rates of mental illness estimated from individual cross-sectional studies, in which people report retrospectively, are much greater than those found in longitudinal studies, in which people report their symptoms closer to the time that they occur (Srole et al., 1978; Murphy et al., 1984). A comparison of estimates from two very similar studies, the 1994 NCS and the 2001–3 NCS-R, also suggests that there has been no systematic upward trend in prevalence. Overall assessments of the cross-cohort literature suggest that the apparent increase in depression in younger generations may primarily reflect poor recall by elderly persons. To the extent that there has been a cross-cohort increase in prevalence, it seems likely to be relatively small.

For children and adolescents treatment and diagnosis rates are increasing rapidly, but considerable uncertainty exists about whether overall rates of mental illnesses are increasing across different generations of children. Several researchers have described the marked rise over the past twenty years in treatment rates for ADHD and depression and mental illnesses more generally. But these changes could be attributable to clinicians' better recognition and training rather than true prevalence increases. Surveys of parents also suggest increasing rates of behavioral problems in their children. But here too the apparent increase might not be in true prevalence, but rather greater openness about mental illness.

Projecting Backward

An alternative way of examining trends in the prevalence of mental illness is to use the most recent surveys to project backward over time. This method assumes that whatever causes mental illness has remained relatively stable, even if the constructs have changed. By examining changes over time in factors correlated with the presence of mental illness, we can assess whether the size of the population of people with mental illness is likely to have changed substantially. A significant problem in this approach, however, is that we know only a few of the factors that predict mental illness.

Epidemiologic studies typically measure race, ethnicity, gender, age, education, income, family structure, and place of residence. The composition of the general population in terms of many of these factors has changed substantially over the past fifty years. As we showed above, the relationship of mental illness to these sociodemographic factors has not changed substantially over this period. We have estimated the correlation between these demographic factors and the prevalence of mental illness at a point in time using a recent, well-conducted survey, the NCS, and applying a standard linear regression analysis. By applying these estimated coefficients to decennial census data, we can generate internally consistent estimates of the size of this population in the past.[11]

We first examined whether readily measurable factors have some power to predict the prevalence of mental illness measured in terms of symptoms or functioning. We examined the predictive power of a set of sociodemographic covariates (including gender, age, race, education, urbanness, and household composition) in the NCS. To exploit the data fully, we included both direct and interaction effects among the factors described above.[12] These sociodemographic covariates explain about 4 percent of variation in symptoms and 10 percent of variation in impairment.

We used these estimates to construct an estimate of the change in the size of the population with mental illness associated with changes in these sociodemographic factors using the 1950 through 1990 U.S. Census (table 2.4). As expected, given the relatively low explanatory power of these covariates with respect to symptoms and impairment, we found only small predicted changes in rates over time. Both symptom and impairment rates peaked in 1980 and have fallen slightly since. We estimate that overall rates of diagnosable mental illnesses rose about two percentage points between 1950 and 1980, from 27 to 29 percent. Because the U.S. population has grown, however, these small changes translate into

TABLE 2.4
Projections of the Number of People Aged 15–54 with Mental Illness

	Percentage with Diagnosis	No. with Diagnosis (millions)	Percentage with Impairment	No. with Impairment (millions)	No. with Serious and Persistent Mental Illness
NCS	28.9	—	6.2	—	—
1950	27.4	23.0	6.1	5.1	1.4
1960	27.5	25.3	6.1	5.6	1.6
1970	28.6	30.3	6.3	6.7	1.8
1980	29.6	37.9	6.6	8.5	2.2
1990	29.0	41.2	6.4	9.1	2.4

NOTE: Projections of number with a diagnosis or impairment are based on regression forecast adjusting for changes in the gender, age, race, education, urbanness, and household composition of the U.S. population. Projections of number with serious and persistent mental illness use a rate of 1.7% of the adult population.

relatively large changes in the absolute number of persons with mental illness. We estimate that the number of people with mental health symptoms (impairment) increased by nearly 80 percent over this period.

We calculated the prevalence of serious mental illness in U.S. households among the adult population by simply taking an average of the prevalence rates in the data sources on severe disability discussed above. We arrived at a prevalence in the adult U.S. household population of 17 per 1,000 persons.

Defining Mental Illness Today

The approximate size of the population with mental illness as a proportion of the full population does not appear to have changed much over the past five decades. In part, however, that stability is a consequence of the coarseness of our measures of mental illness. Those measures include people with a wide range of disorders that generate thoroughly different symptom profiles: people whose ability to function varies from mildly impaired to entirely disabled; people who may prove dangerous to themselves or others; and people who are not a danger to anyone at all. The coarseness of existing measures of mental illness is apparent in the fact that, in our analysis of past studies, neither inclusion nor exclusion of the institutionalized population, whether in psychiatric hospitals, residential treatment facilities, or jails—a group who undoubtedly have very serious illness at extremely elevated rates—had a meaningful effect on our overall population estimates.

Psychiatric epidemiologists continually strive to improve the validity and reliability of the measures they use. But their focus has been on estimating the prevalence of mental illness, broadly defined, in the population. These efforts have yielded estimates that, even when refined, show that one-fifth of the population has some form of mental illness. The extraordinary heterogeneity of the population so defined, however, limits the usefulness of this statistic for policy purposes.

Scientists and philosophers continue to debate the appropriate conceptualization of mental illness. Facing this diverse population, policy analysts must revert to instrumental definitions. Estimates of the size and character of the population with mental illness that are useful for policy making need to take into explicit account the array of policies that affect people with mental illness. These include, for example, policies that affect coverage of treatment for mental illness under private and public insurance plans, policies that address the quality of mental health treatment, policies for funding mental health research, and policies that provide housing and income assistance. Each of these classes of policy—and other classes as well—requires counting a different population.

In most cases, these policy-relevant subpopulations constitute far less than 20 percent of the adult population. In particular, the 20 percent figure does not reflect the number who would require income support, it does not reflect the potential market for any possible pharmacologic treatment, and it does not represent the proportion of an employed population that would likely take advantage of insured mental health services under a parity benefit. A smaller number of precisely measured conditions will be more useful for policy purposes than a broad array of heterogeneous classifications.

Conclusions

Both the range of surveys reviewed and the projections backward based on the NCS suggest that between 15 and 30 percent of the U.S. population had a diagnosable mental illness over a twelve-month period. Although diagnosable illness is concentrated among those with low socioeconomic status, the overall rate of mental illness is not sensitive to changes in this or other population characteristics. Using the NCS to make backward projections, we found that a much smaller fraction of the population, about 5–7 percent, experiences a significant functional impairment at any point. Again, this rate has remained quite steady over time. Finally, about 1.7 percent of the population has a severe and persistent mental illness at any time.

The apparent stability of the prevalence of mental illness over time is important in understanding the role of policy. If the prevalence of illness were changing substantially, observed variations in the use of services might best be ascribed to a changing need for services. Instead, this stability suggests that observed changes in the level and nature of service use over time reflect changes in the demand for and supply of mental health services for a given population. The demand for and supply of mental health services, in turn, are likely to be affected directly and indirectly by changes in mental health policy.

CHAPTER 3

The Evolving Technology of Mental Health Care

The past fifty years have been filled with technological innovations in health care. From the polio vaccine to water fluoridation, from new pharmaceuticals to joint replacement, the benefits of new technologies over the past half century have been staggering. The economist William Nordhaus estimates that during these years the value of improved health from new technologies was roughly equal to the growth in the U.S. gross domestic product (Nordhaus, 2003). Improvements in treatment technologies are likely to be a particularly significant contributor to well-being for people with any disabling condition, including mental illness.

For some diseases, technological innovation has been nothing short of revolutionary. Smallpox, polio, and measles have been eradicated in the wealthiest nations through the development and administration of vaccines. Consider, as well, the near elimination of Hansen's disease (also known as leprosy), a chronic, disabling condition that, like mental illness, had its own dedicated provider systems in 1950. Mental illness has not been as fortunate. Most of its treatments remain "halfway technologies" that manage symptoms but do not alter the underlying disease (Thomas, 1974). For the most part, we have not improved our ability to cure or prevent these diseases over the past half century. Yet there have been substantial improvements in relieving symptoms of mental illness, and they have contributed importantly to the well-being of people with mental illness. This chapter examines technological developments in the treatment of mental health problems over the past fifty years.

We compared "then" (the 1950s and 1960s) to "now" by looking closely at the best available treatment technologies at each point in time—the technological frontier.[1] We did this by comparing today's practice guidelines with the scientific literature of the past and two prominent psychiatric textbooks from earlier eras: the *American Handbook of Psychiatry* (1959), by Silvano Arieti, and the *Comprehensive Textbook of Psychiatry* (1967), by Alfred Freedman, Harold Kaplan, and Helen

Kaplan. To analyze the nature of treatment advances, we have also drawn on FDA records, comparative clinical trials,[2] and histories of psychiatric treatments. Our focus is on schizophrenia, depression, anxiety disorders, and ADHD, which collectively account for most mental illness.

Technological changes may extend the technological frontier by providing new treatments or by improving knowledge about existing treatments. Improved knowledge about existing treatments may lead to exnovation (removal from practice) of existing technologies that turn out to be harmful or to new uses for existing technologies.[3] These too serve to extend the "best practice" frontier. Some important innovations, however, do not advance the technological frontier. Rather, they enhance the ability of providers and consumers to reach the existing frontier. In our discussion below, we group innovations into three categories.

Efficacy advance—a new treatment dominates the best treatments in the earlier era because of its superiority in reducing target symptoms and advances the technological frontier.

Exnovation—an old treatment that was ineffective or harmful is no longer, or less frequently, offered as a result of new knowledge, which likewise advances the frontier.

Practice advance—a new treatment is no more efficacious than the old one, and so it does not extend the frontier; yet is safer, more tolerable, or easier to prescribe or use.

Most assessments of technology focus on the state of the technological frontier. Innovations that extend the frontier are very important, but the study of technological advance suggests that the effect of a technology also depends on the ease with which it can be diffused. The long history of inventions that were "before their time"—consider Leonardo da Vinci's helicopter in the 1500s or Charles Babbage's computer in the 1800s—demonstrates the central importance of diffusion. A recent survey of technological change noted that "it is diffusion rather than invention or innovation that ultimately determines the pace of economic growth and the rate of change of productivity" (Hall and Khan, 2003). Advances in practice facilitate this diffusion.

In medicine the importance of different types of innovation is likely to depend on the policy context. In a system dominated by a small number of specialist providers, where consumers have few choices over care, efficacy advances and exnovation are likely to be most important because the care delivered depends critically on the state of knowledge. By contrast, in a fragmented and pluralistic system, advances that make it easier to deliver and tolerate treatment may be more important than efficacy advances in improving the quality of care that people actually receive. Of course, a cure for any mental illness would be a tremendously valuable efficacy advance regardless of the design of the mental health system.

Schizophrenia

Our measure of today's technological frontier for the treatment of schizophrenia is drawn from the schizophrenia Patient Outcomes Research Team (PORT), a federally funded research project. The PORT developed thirty recommendations structured around several treatment modalities: pharmacotherapy, psychotherapy, family intervention, vocational rehabilitation, and assertive community treatment (Lehman and Steinwachs, 1998). These have been consolidated into nine key recommendations by Lehman (1999), reported in table 3.1. For ease of comparison with practices of the 1950s and 1960s, we focused on advances in medications and psychotherapy. We find that today's more complex treatments and combinations are new arrangements of treatment elements that have long existed.

The History of Medications

The first wave of pharmacologic innovation for schizophrenia occurred in the 1950s, and it led to enormous breakthroughs in treatment (table 3.2). The advent

TABLE 3.1
Recommended Treatments for Schizophrenia

1. Antipsychotic medication for acute symptoms

2. Antipsychotic dose for acute symptoms equivalent to 300–1,000 mg chlorpromazine per day

3. Antipsychotic medication for maintenance treatment

4. Maintenance antipsychotic dose equivalent to 300–600 mg chlorpromazine per day

5. Anti-Parkinsonian medication for side effects

6. Antidepressant medication for depressed patients

7. Psychotherapy or counseling

8. Family and educational support

9. Vocational rehabilitation

SOURCE: Data from Lehman and Steinwachs, 1998; Lehman, 1999.

of the first generation of antipsychotic drugs was one of several factors contributing to the release of patients from state mental hospitals. The enduring significance of these drugs from the 1950s and 1960s is evident in the fact that they still remain frontline treatments in today's PORT recommendations.

Chlorpromazine was the first medication to take the psychiatric world by storm, heralding the modern era of biological psychiatry. A Parisian surgeon, Henri Laborit, who had been searching for an anesthetic, discovered that the drug dramatically calmed patients instead of anesthetizing them. Immediately grasping the drug's psychiatric potential, Laborit found that chlorpromazine alleviated hallucinations and delusions in psychiatric patients. It was introduced in Europe in 1952 by the French drug company Rhone-Poulenc. Two years later the drug was introduced in the United States by the drugmaker Smith, Kline and French under the brand name Thorazine (Shen, 1999). Although some small clinical trials of chlorpromazine were conducted during the 1950s, the first large-scale trial, and the most robust of its kind (a double-blind, placebo-controlled clinical trial), was not published until 1960 (Casey, Bennett, et al., 1960). In 1958 an analogue of chlorpromazine was introduced into the market, the drug haloperidol (under the brand name Haldol). By the mid-1960s a large-scale, placebo-controlled trial was completed, again with promising outcomes (Shen, 1999).

New developments appear in textbooks after a time lag, mostly because of delays in publication and in diffusion of information. The *American Handbook of Psychiatry*, published in 1959, does not capture the reported successes of chlorpromazine. Instead, the textbook describes psychotherapy as the "treatment of choice." "One finds, first of all, marked disagreements as to treatment of choice. My own marked preference, in the average case, is psychotherapy, although many authors and practitioners do not share this point of view. My 'bias' is based on the belief that . . . psychotherapy tends to (1) remove the basic conflicts which led to the disorder,

TABLE 3.2
Chronology of Antipsychotic Drugs

1952–54	Chlorpromazine marketed in United States
1958	Haloperidol introduced in United States
1959	Clozapine introduced in Europe
1975	Molindone introduced in United States
1989	Clozapine introduced in United States
1994	Risperidone introduced in United States
1996	Olanzapine introduced in United States
1997	Quetiapine introduced in United States

(2) correct the psychopathologic patterns, and (3) permit the regenerative psychological powers of the organism to regain the lost ground" (Arieti, 1959, 493).

By 1967, when the *Comprehensive Textbook of Psychiatry* (1967) was published, chlorpromazine and similar drugs were described as treatment breakthroughs. The doses recommended for chlorpromazine are remarkably consistent with those promulgated more than thirty years later by the schizophrenia PORT (300 to 1,000 mg). Thus, by the 1960s the administration of chlorpromazine for the treatment of acute symptoms of schizophrenia was widely understood and recommended.

Today's PORT recommendations also deal with management and dosing of antipsychotic drugs for maintenance treatment to control symptoms and reduce relapses. Interestingly, ideas about maintenance treatment were advanced in the early 1960s. In his Bampton Lectures at Columbia University in 1965, the preeminent psychiatrist Robert Felix, who had been the director of the National Institute of Mental Health (NIMH), hailed the importance of managing severely mentally ill patients in the community using maintenance doses of antipsychotic medication (Felix, 1965). Although controlled trials of maintenance doses were not published until the late 1970s, the 1967 *Textbook* recommended specific doses of maintenance medications that are similar to today's doses.

Traditional antipsychotic drugs such as chlorpromazine and haloperidol produce a variety of side effects. By far the most prevalent and debilitating is extrapyramidal syndrome (EPS), a condition marked by rigidity, tremor, and motor inertia (akinesia). Though EPS was recognized as early as 1954, documentation of its widespread prevalence came in 1961, with research showing that 40 percent of patients were affected (Shen, 1999). EPS was so widely regarded as a problem that by 1967 the *Comprehensive Textbook* recommended a separate medication, an anti-Parkinsonian drug, expressly to combat it. Anti-Parkinsonian medications are still recommended today. The consequences of EPS were documented as early as 1978 by a study finding lower treatment compliance rates and higher relapse rates for patients experiencing those side effects (Van Putten and May, 1978).

The new generation of so-called atypical antipsychotic medications marketed in the late 1980s and 1990s—including, clozapine, olanzapine, quetiapine, and risperidone—are, in general, comparable to traditional antipsychotics in efficacy. The significant advantage of the new generation of drugs is relief from EPS, which is often critical to patients' willingness to start and stay with treatment. The reduction in EPS with one or more of the new generation of antipsychotic medications has been borne out in at least two meta-analyses, large studies that quantitatively pooled results across multiple previously published clinical trials (Rosenheck et al., 1997; Geddes et al., 2000; Leucht et al., 2003). A lower rate of

EPS symptoms translates into a greater likelihood of patients' staying on the drug (Geddes et al., 2000; Lieberman et al., 2003).

There has been heated debate about whether the new generation of antipsychotic drugs also represents a general efficacy advance. A few clinical trials have found the new generation generally superior to the traditional ones, but the trials are small and, some experts argue, poorly designed (Geddes et al., 2000; Leucht et al., 2003). Looming over the debate is the considerably higher cost of the new generation of drugs.

For some 30 percent of all schizophrenic patients who are treatment refractory (they exhibit a lack of response to three trials of antipsychotic medications from at least two different classes), clozapine represents an efficacy advance. A double-blind clinical trial in the mid-1980s showing that clozapine was the most efficacious treatment for treatment-resistant patients (Kane et al., 1988) led to clozapine's approval by the FDA in 1989 (Shen, 1999).[4] The PORT study also supports the use of clozapine for these patients (Lehmann et al., 1998). For treatment-resistant patients, clozapine represents both an efficacy advance and a practice advance.

Exnovation

Arieti's 1959 textbook had recommend psychotherapy as first-line therapy for schizophrenia. In the 1960s psychodynamic psychotherapies came under fierce scrutiny, although the first stirrings of dissent had taken place a decade earlier. In 1952 the psychologist Hans Eysenck, after evaluating twenty-four published studies, concluded in a landmark paper that none of the psychotherapies performed better than chance (Eysenck, 1952). By the 1960s psychodynamic therapies began to be rejected in favor of biological psychiatry and more evidence-based forms of psychotherapy. The shift in standards of care is captured in the eight-year interval between publication of the 1959 *Handbook* and the 1967 *Comprehensive Textbook*. The former, which advocates psychotherapy as the treatment of choice for schizophrenia, traces its position back to Freud. "Freud's concept that the libido of the schizophrenic is withdrawn from an external object, making it impossible to establish transference, for many years discouraged therapists from attempting to treat patients with this disorder. Actually, psychoanalysis opened the road to the psychotherapy of schizophrenia after some modifications of the classic method were made" (Arieti, 1959, 494).

The 1967 *Comprehensive Textbook*, while still retaining some of the elements of psychodynamic therapy, also emphasized the importance of present behavior, the development of a relationship with the therapist to ease anxiety, and the creation of hope. The shift to what is now called "supportive psychotherapy," used exclusively in conjunction with medications, was propelled in 1968 with publication of a pioneering clinical trial, which found that patients treated with drugs fared the best, whereas those treated with only psychodynamic therapies fared no better than controls (May, 1968). Other studies in the late 1960s and early 1970s found that supportive counseling in combination with antipsychotic medication significantly reduced the likelihood of relapse in schizophrenia (Hogarty and Goldberg, 1973).

Today individual and group psychotherapy is essential as an adjunct to medication, according to the PORT. Also spelled out by the PORT study are the ingredients of psychotherapy—namely, support, education, and development of behavioral and cognitive skills. The recommendations explicitly caution against the use of Freudian-inspired psychodynamic psychotherapies, which are characterized as harmful and expensive (Lehman and Steinwachs, 1998). The PORT states flatly that "individual and group psychotherapy adhering to a psychodynamic model (defined as therapies that use interpretation of unconscious material and focus on transference and regression) should not be used in the treatment of persons with schizophrenia. . . . There is a consensus that psychotherapy that promotes regression and psychotic transference can be harmful to persons with schizophrenia."

The 1960s also saw the demise of a host of ineffective, inhumane, and outright harmful therapies. The list includes hydrotherapy, insulin shock therapy, and psychosurgery (Shorter, 1997). Some 20,000 people underwent psychosurgery from 1936 to 1951, before the introduction of antipsychotic medications (Donelly, 1980). The antipsychotics were so efficacious that they also replaced earlier pharmacotherapy, dominated by barbiturates and reserpine. The civil rights movement also played a role in the exnovation of therapies as psychiatric patients began to assert their rights.

Psychiatric educators did not greet the shift away from the somatic therapies with universal praise. The *Comprehensive Textbook* (1967) stated that the rare use of insulin shock was regrettable because "there was a definite need for the continuation of this treatment." Its demise was attributed to the difficulty and hazards of its administration. The *Textbook* also viewed psychosurgery in a relatively positive light, noting that it "has greatly augmented the hope that one day our accumulated knowledge of the relationship between brain, personality, and mental disorder will constitute an exact science" (chap. 35). Nevertheless, by the mid-1960s many treatments that had been quite prevalent in the late 1940s and 1950s were largely obsolete.

In summary, clinical gains in the treatment of schizophrenia in the earlier part of the period from 1950 to 2000 included a high rate of exnovation, as many inappropriate, ineffective, or inhumane treatments were discontinued as a consequence of new knowledge and new attitudes. Since 1960 there have been several advances in antipsychotic medications. To a large extent, the main benefit of the newer atypical antipsychotic medications is that they are practice advances—they are easier to tolerate and to administer.[5] The development of these medications was coincident with a shift in the context of treatment for schizophrenia—from more controlled institutional settings staffed by a limited number of specialists to community settings where patients faced more choices of treatment, provider, and setting.

Depression

In 1993 a panel of experts assembled by a relatively new government agency, created in 1989 to improve the quality of health care, developed practice guidelines for depression, the first developed for a psychiatric disorder (AHCPR, 1993). Another set of practice guidelines was issued under the auspices of the American Psychiatric Association (APA, 1993). Both sets of guidelines feature, for the acute phase of treatment, two classes of frontline medications (the selective serotonin reuptake inhibitors [SSRIs] and tricyclic antidepressants [TCAs]) and several forms of psychotherapy. Also highlighted are preferred methods for the continuation or maintenance phase of treatment. For all phases of treatment, the guidelines give dose ranges for medication as well as duration and frequency of psychotherapy.

The History of Medications

Much was known about acute-phase treatment of depression in the 1950s and 1960s. That era saw the introduction of monoamine oxidase inhibitors (MAOIs) and TCAs (table 3.3). For both classes of medication, the general dose ranges and duration proposed then still hold. In today's guidelines, TCAs remain as frontline treatments. On the other hand, the MAOIs have been moved to the second tier because of the potential for fatal interactions with other medications and the requirement to avoid certain foods with their use (AHCPR, 1993; APA, 1993).

As early as 1959 the *Handbook* by Arieti noted that the MAOI iproniazid was likely to be helpful and perhaps as effective for treating depression as electrocon-

TABLE 3.3
Time Line of Treatments for Depression

1956	TCA Tofranil (imipramine) appears
1959	MAOIs Marplan and Nardil introduced
1961	TCA amitriptyline introduced
1963	TCA nortriptyline introduced
1967	TCA protiptyline introduced; first mentions of interpersonal psychotherapy, behavioral therapy
1974	First mention of cognitive therapy
1975	Generic imipramine marketed
1976	Generic amitriptyline marketed
1982	HCA[a] trazodone introduced
1986	HCA buproprion introduced
1988	SSRI fluoxetine introduced
1992	SSRI sertraline introduced
1993	SSRI paroxetine introduced
1994	SNRI[b] venlafaxine introduced

[a]HCA: heterocyclic antidepressant.
[b]SNRI: serotonin-norepinephrine reuptake inhibitor.

vulsive therapy. Several studies later confirmed what clinicians had noticed in the early 1950s: iproniazid's action against tuberculosis seemed also to improve patients' mood. The first clinical study of the TCA imipramine in 1961 found it efficacious (Angst, 1961). The study also indicated that positive responses to imipramine carried over from one episode to future episodes. Some years later several controlled studies showed that depression relapse rates fell by about half as a result of TCA treatment (Carlsson et al., 1969; Morris and Beck, 1974). The early studies also determined that TCAs were associated with treatment failures that were due to intolerance of side effects, inadequate doses, and insufficient duration of treatment.

Reflecting the accumulating knowledge at the time, the 1967 *Textbook* detailed how imipramine should be used for the treatment of depression, including the ranges of effective doses and the timing of initial responses and maximum response. It also characterized MAOIs and the TCA amitriptyline as helpful. The *Textbook* suggested that weaning patients from drugs should begin after four to six weeks of treatment. This is just a little briefer than today's guidelines for acute-phase treatment. Some references were made in 1967 to relapse prevention, but there is little discussion of what is now considered either continuation- or maintenance-phase treatment.

The advent of the SSRIs, beginning with Prozac in 1988, transformed the treatment of depression; these drugs entered both the medical mainstream, through their widespread use by primary care providers, and the popular culture, with Peter Kramer's best-selling book in 1993, *Listening to Prozac.*

The therapeutic gains of SSRIs represent more of a practice advance than an efficacy advance. Studies tend to find that SSRIs and TCAs are of comparable efficacy. Yet the SSRIs are safer, better tolerated by patients, and easier for clinicians to prescribe because they have an uncomplicated dosing regimen and they pose less danger from overdose (US DHHS, 1999). Three meta-analyses of the 1990s that compared SSRIs with TCAs found them to be of comparable efficacy. But SSRI treatment had significantly lower rates of patient dropout during clinical studies (Song et al., 1993; Le Pen et al., 1994; Montgomery et al., 1994; Anderson and Tomenson, 1995). Similarly, a meta-analysis found that the overall dropout rate from treatment with SSRIs was 10 percent lower than with TCAs. In the same analysis dropouts specifically due to side effects, as opposed to other reasons, were 25 percent lower with SSRIs (Anderson and Tomenson, 1995; Trindade et al., 1998; Peretti et al., 2000). Thus, the evidence is clear that SSRIs represent an important practice advance in terms of safety, tolerability, and ease of prescribing.

As in the case of schizophrenia, this innovation occurred in part because of the shifting practice context regarding treatment of depression. Epidemiologic findings from the mid-1980s had suggested that primary care was the setting where most people with depression sought care (Regier et al., 1993; US DHHS, 1999). The trend toward increased primary care treatment of depression was further propelled by the growth in managed care, which encourages primary care as a cheaper alternative to specialty care. This shift in practice made primary care the target of the first set of depression practice guidelines (AHCPR, 1993). Practice advances that made care easier to deliver were essential if primary care doctors were to effectively treat the many people with depression who sought care in this setting.

The History of Psychotherapy

In the 1959 *Handbook* psychodynamic psychotherapy was the main strategy for depression treatment (Arieti, 1959). Yet Eysenck's 1952 landmark review, and later others, concluded that these therapies offered no benefits over the natural course of illness (Levitt, 1963; Eysenck, 1965; Parloff, 1984). As evidence mounted, the 1967 *Comprehensive Textbook* broke ranks with the earlier textbook. It asserted that probing into unconscious factors—the goal of psychodynamic therapies— was not helpful and might make patients more anxious. It noted that therapy should be aimed at combating depressive ideas and interpreting the illness in physical terms. Another goal was to encourage daily activities that a patient could achieve. For milder forms of depression, psychotherapy was viewed as the treatment of choice. Behavior therapy is mentioned as a new treatment designed to change overt behavior. Interpersonal therapy and cognitive therapy first appeared in the psychiatric literature during the late 1960s and early 1970s. Controlled studies of their efficacy were reported by the mid-1970s (Klerman et al., 1974; Beck, 1976; Rush et al., 1977). These therapies, involving twelve to sixteen weeks of treatment, were shown to produce significant clinical gains. Studies from the mid-1970s showed that psychotherapy in combination with pharmacotherapy had a more than additive effect on treatment outcomes (Luborsky et al., 1975).

Because of the strong evidence of their efficacy, cognitive behavioral therapy and interpersonal therapy are the two psychotherapies recommended by today's guidelines (APA, 1993). Cognitive behavioral therapy strives to reduce symptoms by challenging and reversing irrational beliefs and distorted attitudes, whereas interpersonal therapy concentrates on losses, role disputes and transitions, social skill deficits, and other interpersonal issues. Both types of psychotherapy are considered as effective as medications.

Exnovation

Psychodynamic therapies, at their height in the 1940s, began to ebb in the 1960s. The confluence of new pharmacologic treatments, evidence of weak efficacy, and the high costs for therapy of extended duration made these therapies relatively unattractive (Shorter, 1997; Dolnick, 1998).

Exnovation of electroconvulsive therapy (ECT) took a more unexpected route. After its introduction in 1934, ECT was hailed as a breakthrough in treatment for depression, schizophrenia, and other psychiatric maladies. Over time, though, it gained notoriety from unsafe and sometimes inhumane administration. Reports emerged of patients breaking limbs and fracturing vertebrate as their bodies gyrated on the operating table (Shorter, 1997). In the 1950s and 1960s ECT made headlines as a rallying point for psychiatry's critics. Its use plummeted. Reflecting the decline, the 1959 *Handbook* recommended ECT only for psychotic depression, not for neurotic depression. Over the years the medical profession made safety enhancements, especially in the use of anesthesia. Buoyed during the next decades by research firmly establishing its safety, efficacy, and quick onset of action, ECT eventually regained frontline status in the treatment of the most severe forms of depression (ACHPR, 1993). ECT also gained acceptance for use in depressed older adults on the rationale that they are slower to respond to and less able to tolerate antidepressant medication (NIH Consensus Development Panel on Depression in Late Life, 1992).

Anxiety Disorders

The treatment of anxiety disorders has changed greatly over the past fifty years. The mainstays of anxiety treatment in the 1950s are now largely obsolete: psychodynamic therapies and the tranquilizer meprobamate, or Miltown, which predated Valium as the first blockbuster psychiatric drug. In its heyday there were claims that meprobamate was taken by one in twenty Americans, many of whom probably had very mild anxieties (Shorter, 1997).

The modern era of pharmacotherapy for anxiety disorders began in 1964 with the publication of the results of a clinical trial of the TCA imipramine. That trial provided the first evidence that an antidepressant could be efficacious for panic disorder (Klein, 1964). The trial was so pivotal that it led to the creation of panic disorder as a new diagnostic entity, formally recognized in the DSM by 1980 (Katon, 1993). The success of imipramine in the 1960s unleashed a wave of research applying other antidepressants then available—TCAs and MAOIs—to the treatment of other anxiety disorders. These classes of antidepressants still are used today for various anxiety disorders, albeit as second-line treatments. As in the case of depression, the first-line medications—the SSRIs—have superior safety and tolerability profiles over the older classes, yet roughly comparable efficacy (APA, 1998). Thus, since 1964, practice advances have constituted the bulk of innovation in the treatment of most anxiety disorders.

Obsessive-Compulsive Disorder

The treatment of obsessive-compulsive disorder (OCD), alone in the class of anxiety disorders, represents a case of innovation in efficacy. None of today's standard therapies for OCD—neither pharmacotherapies nor psychotherapies—was available fifty years ago.

Today's practice guidelines for OCD were developed in 1997 through an expert consensus process (March et al., 1997). The guidelines call solely for cognitive behavioral therapy (CBT) for milder cases of OCD, or CBT in combination with an SSRI for more severe cases (table 3.4). The second-line medication (after failure of two to three SSRIs) is clomipramine, which is a TCA with some SSRI-like pharmacologic properties, that is, inhibition of serotonin reuptake. In terms of psychotherapy, the guidelines specify use of a particular type of CBT with

TABLE 3.4

Expert Consensus Guidelines: Obsessive-Compulsive Disorder

Medication	Dose (mg/day)
First-line treatment	
SSRI (fluvoxamine, fluoxeine, sertraline, paroxetine)	50–200
Second-line treatment	
clomipramine after 2–3 failed SSRIs venlafaxine	200
Medication management: taper after 1–2 years	

Psychotherapy	Duration	Frequency
Cognitive behavioral therapy, consisting of: exposure/response prevention cognitive therapy	13–20 weeks	1/week

Continuation/maintenance for 2–4 relapses	Frequency
Medication dosed at acute level	1–6 months
Medication management visits	

SOURCE: Data from March et al., 1997.

two components: exposure/response prevention, a particular form of behavior therapy, mixed with cognitive therapy.

The History of Medications

The mainstays of pharmacotherapy in the 1990s—clomipramine and SSRIs—were not yet available in the 1950s and 1960s. In the United States the modern era of pharmacotherapy for OCD began in the late 1980s with success in several controlled clinical trials of the TCA clomipramine (Leonard et al., 1989), whose benefit for OCD had been noted decades earlier by European physicians when they noticed that depressed, suicidal patients—who also happened to have obsessions—had both their depression and obsessions eased with the drug (Dolnick, 1998). By 1967 clomipramine was successfully tested for OCD in an open clinical trial in Europe (Lopez-Ibor and Fernandez-Cordoba, 1967). But it did not reach the U.S. market until 1989, when the FDA approved it for OCD. After several intervening years, large-scale U.S. epidemiology studies revealed that OCD was not as rare as the field believed. Clomipramine's efficacy is equivalent, or arguably superior, to that of the SSRIs (Todorov et al., 2000). But clomipramine carries greater adverse effects, including cardiac and anticholinergic effects (e.g., dry mouth, sweating, constipation, and significant weight gain) (March et al., 1997).

In the 1950s and 1960s textbooks referred to OCD as "obsessive-compulsive reaction" or "obsessive-compulsive neurosis."[6] The 1959 *Handbook* describes several psychodynamic therapies, but it makes no mention of pharmacotherapy. In 1967 the *Textbook* reflected continued support for psychodynamic therapy, yet it was more explicit about the *lack* of pharmacotherapies for OCD: "There are no drugs that have a specific action on the obsessive-compulsive symptoms themselves, although the use of sedatives and tranquilizers as an adjunct to psychotherapy may be helpful in cases where anxiety is excessive" (Freedman and Kaplan, 1967). The *Textbook* stated that antidepressant medications of the era, the TCAs and MAOIs, had "no direct effect" on obsessions and compulsions. This was later borne out in controlled clinical trials, beginning in the 1980s, which found that TCAs lacking serotonin effects did not work as well as clomipramine (and SSRIs) for OCD (Leonard et al., 1989; Pigott and Seay, 1999).

The History of Psychotherapy

Fifty years ago, Freudian therapies for OCD predominated. Freudians viewed obsessions and compulsions as being rooted in the anal phase of infant psychosexual development. The theory gave rise to psychodynamic therapies that could shed light on infantile conflicts in order to discharge so-called repressed rages. In 1959 the *Handbook* described psychodynamic therapies of three different varieties, only one of which—labeled "reconstructive treatment"—was judged by the author as "the method of choice." Still, the *Handbook* admitted that results with this preferred method were only "fair to good" for the average patient, but they were "hopeless" for severe patients. After describing the two other therapies, the *Handbook* observed, "As to the merit of each school's treatment of obsessional behavior . . . one would have to be familiar with each school's technique through practical experience. To my regret, I am not. Unfortunately every psychoanalytic school speaks its own language. Reduction of this Babel to one tongue has not yet been attempted" (Arieti, 1959).

The 1967 *Textbook* lent lukewarm support to psychodynamic therapy explicitly because of the absence of controlled studies and ignorance about the natural history of OCD. The *Textbook* also devoted a paragraph to some new types of behavior therapy, yet it concluded that it was too early to determine their efficacy. The 1967 *Textbook* made no mention of any type of exposure therapy.

Not until the late 1970s and 1980s was research published in support of exposure/response prevention (E/RP) (Foster and Eisler, 2001). E/RP reduces obsessions by repeatedly exposing patients to the feared stimulus (e.g., germs) and by having them explicitly refrain from compulsive behaviors, whether rituals (e.g., hand washing) or avoidance behavior. Cognitive therapy works to reduce patients' catastrophic thinking and heightened sense of personal responsibility and to challenge faulty assumptions underlying obsessions (March et al., 1997). The melding of E/RP with cognitive therapy was not even mentioned until the 1995 edition of the *Textbook*. Today it is the gold standard for psychotherapy.

Exnovation

Exnovation occurred for three OCD treatments—ECT, psychoanalysis, and psychosurgery—but much exnovation had already taken place before publication of the 1959 *Handbook*. ECT was not mentioned in the text even though it had been used for OCD since the 1930s. The 1967 *Textbook* was more unequivocal in its denunciation, declaring ECT to have "no direct effect on obsessions and compulsions."

The 1959 *Handbook* questioned the value of some psychodynamic therapies for OCD. Similarly, the 1967 *Textbook* was skeptical of psychodynamic therapy because of the lack of research, but it did not formally pronounce it to be ineffective until several decades later, in the 1995 edition. For the first time the message was unambiguous: "Traditional psychodynamic psychotherapy is not considered an effective treatment for obsessions and rituals" (Kaplan and Sadock, 1995).

Attention Deficit Hyperactivity Disorder

There has also been innovation in the treatment of mental illnesses in children, most notably in attention deficit hyperactivity disorder (ADHD). ADHD has been recognized as a disorder among children for more than a century. Ritalin and several other stimulant medications were introduced as early as 1956, which ranks them among the first available medications for any psychiatric disorder. Treatment has evolved since then but its trajectory charts a familiar course: as with most other disorders, the past half century of treatment for ADHD has witnessed practice advances and exnovation rather than advances in treatment efficacy.

The History of Medications

ADHD as been variously labeled minimal brain dysfunction, hyperactivity syndrome, and attention deficit disorder; its basic description harkens back to the English physician George Still's 1902 description in the *Lancet*. In Still's words, affected children were "passionate, deviant, spiteful, and lacking inhibitory volition." Because the children had been raised by "good" parents—in fact, he had excluded children reared "poorly" according to norms of his era—Still speculated that a biological or genetic defect was the cause. The idea of a biological defect appealed to the American psychologist William James, whose interest helped to launch a discussion of causation that lasted for the next several decades (Hallowell and Ratey, 1994). In 1937 the pediatrician Charles Bradley serendipitously discovered that a stimulant helped to reduce hyperkinetic activity and make children more compliant (Bradley, 1937). The idea of a stimulant calming children down was surprising and counterintuitive, but, through a series of studies, Bradley and others were able to document its efficacy (Molitch and Eccles, 1937; Bradley and Bowen, 1940), despite the fact that the drug's working to ease ADHD still remains a mystery. Their studies also showed that children who were given stimulants improved their academic performance and reduced their disruptive behavior. Once these results were repeated in the 1950s, and the stimulant Ritalin was approved by the FDA, a new era of treatment was launched.

Today, some fifty years later, stimulants for ADHD are the most widely prescribed psychotropic drugs for children. In the past fifteen years alone, use is estimated to have increased two- to sixfold (Zito et al., 2000). Its use is so pervasive that the *New Yorker* magazine featured on the cover of its back-to-school issue a cartoon with the "three Rs" inscribed on the blackboard as "readin, ritin, Ritalin." Fueling the surge in use is ADHD's migration to the mainstream of medicine, as progressively more primary care physicians became comfortable prescribing it. From 1990 to 1993, for example, ADHD-related visits to primary care providers increased from 1.6 to 4.2 million per year (Swanson et al., 1995). Stimulants are featured in today's core treatment recommendations for ADHD by the American Academy of Pediatrics (2001) and the American Academy of Child and Adolescent Psychiatry (Dulcan et al., 1997). Dosage levels have changed little over the years.

Practice advances have helped to move stimulants to primary care and catapult their usage. For more than fifty years, three distinct amphetamine-type stimulants formed the treatment arsenal.[7] They were found superior to caffeine and other stimulant agents, and all were easily absorbed and fast-acting. If some children did not respond to one of the stimulants, they might respond to another—and thus treatment options expanded. The stimulants' short duration of action, lasting a matter of hours, however, made dosing a problem. During the 1990s pharmaceutical companies introduced several long-acting forms of the same medications. Two or three doses could now be compressed into one dose. Instead of requiring a dose before school and again at lunch, children need take only one morning dose. These advantages proved highly attractive, for they multiplied consumer choices, diminished the stigma of children being labeled by their schoolmates, and reduced costs of administering medications.

In 2003 a new class of agent, atomoxetine, was released for ADHD treatment. For the first time, a nonstimulant entered the market, one whose mechanism of action is closely related to SSRI antidepressants. When efficacy was compared head-to-head, the benefits of atomoxetine were found to be similar to those of stimulants (Kratochvil et al., 2002). Atomoxetine is a practice advance. Its reduced side effects make it easier for children to tolerate (Kratochvil et al., 2002). Moreover, atomoxetine lacks addiction potential. For years news stories exposed the black market for stimulants, focusing on college students grinding up tablets to snort the powder as they crammed for exams. The stimulants' addiction potential led to restrictions on their availability imposed under the Controlled Substances Act. Lacking addiction potential, atomoxetine is not classified as a controlled substance, so it is more convenient to obtain. Refills can be phoned into pharmacies and samples can be provided to physicians' offices—major advantages over the stimulants.

Several other psychotropic drugs have been used to treat ADHD. TCAs are among the most widely studied. Several investigators noted their efficacy among youth completing clinical trials (Spencer et al., 1994), but it appears that as many as half of all subjects in those studies dropped out because of significant side effects. The potential toxicity associated with TCA overdose also makes some clinicians reluctant to use such drugs. Thus, TCAs are unlikely to be employed for ADHD. Other investigators have considered the newer SSRI antidepressants as possible agents for ADHD when stimulants fail or are unacceptable. The NIH Consensus Conference on ADHD (NIH Consensus Statement, 1998), however, failed to find any evidence of significant improvement in ADHD with these agents. (These same conclusions were reached by Saccar and others twenty years before, when they encouraged others to abandon use of nonstimulant agents [Saccar, 1978].)

The History of Psychotherapy and Other Treatments

During the first half of the twentieth century, youths with ADHD were treated through minimal-stimulation classrooms. The prevailing notion was that brain abnormalities led to involuntary responses to stimuli, and so patients were placed in low-stimuli environments. Prognosis was considered poor.

As awareness of efficacy mounted, the stimulants and various forms of psychotherapy were added to the low-stimuli classrooms in the 1960s, after which special classrooms ceased to be recommended for the treatment of ADHD. It is not clear how much or how often such special classrooms were used. Before the 1950s, when ADHD was seen as an organic brain lesion, psychotherapy does not seem to have had a prominent role. During the 1970s, however, the child's immediate environment was hailed as key to causation. At first environmental food allergies were emphasized. Some physicians claimed that allergies to certain dyes and chemicals in food might cause ADHD. Although this theory was popular with the press and parent groups, in 1980 the National Advisory Committee on Hyperkinesis and Food Additives, reviewing the evidence, found the claims unsupported. A decade later similar concerns were voiced about sugar. The 1998 NIH Consensus Conference found no evidence to support restricting sugar.

Psychotherapists suggested that chemicals and diet were not at fault as much as the immediate social environment of the child. These therapists fell into two camps. The first camp, drawn from the ranks of psychoanalysts, believed that excessively rigid and intolerant parents brought on ADHD by conditioning children to increase their activity level. Today's treatment recommendations from major organizations no longer include psychoanalysis, so its decline represents an exnovation.

The second camp recommended the behavioral therapies that continue today. These include both parent training and classroom management techniques. Although these interventions were effective when compared to placebo, they did not achieve results as robust as stimulants had. Still, many clinicians and most guideline recommendations include some component of behavioral therapy in combination with stimulant medication. A landmark clinical trial of ADHD treatment for nearly six hundred children over a fourteen-month period found that stimulants, alone or in combination with behavioral interventions, achieved significantly better outcomes for children than behavioral interventions alone (Jensen et al., 2001).

What is remarkable about this study is that the treatments being compared—stimulants and behavior therapy—were introduced during a burst of innovation from the 1950s to 1970s. The innovative features being studied were not the therapies per se, but their refinements and their combination—all the hallmarks of practice advances. And not even under remotest consideration, when the clinical trial was designed, were the list of treatments that had fallen by the wayside over the previous fifty years—the special classrooms, the diet restrictions, and the psychoanalysts blaming rigid and controlling parents.

Conclusions

The mental health system's capacity for effective treatment is substantially greater now than it was a half century ago. The choices of efficacious treatment have improved owing to three interrelated types of innovation: efficacy advances, practice advances, and exnovation (table 3.5). Advances in efficacy led the way in the earliest years of this treatment revolution (1950–70), and they were followed by new treatments of similar efficacy that offered significant advantages in terms of practice. Older, less efficacious, and unsafe treatments were discontinued through exnovation. The overall result is a wider array of efficacious treatment options and the expansion of mental health treatment in primary care.

Today's practice guidelines for some of the most prevalent and disabling mental disorders—schizophrenia, depression, and ADHD—still include the blockbuster medications introduced in the 1950s and 1960s.[8] With the exception of treatments for obsessive compulsive disorder, most new treatments were not so superior in efficacy for such a broad range of patients that they completely eliminated earlier ones.

Exnovation has also played a central role in improving the menu of treatment options. Psychoanalysis was replaced by newer therapies for all major disorders. For schizophrenia, the breadth of exnovation was astonishing, as psychoanalysis, psychosurgery, insulin shock therapy, and other ineffective, unsafe, or inhumane therapies were superseded by new treatments. Benzodiazepines and tranquilizers, once touted as panaceas for minor anxieties, were phased out or prescribed much more judiciously to prevent abuse or dependence.

Technological innovation occurs within an institutional context. In mental health there are three such contexts: academic research, pharmaceutical industry research, and practitioner innovation. The goal of grant-funded academic research is usually to push forward the technological frontier. The structure of the clinical trial, the research gold standard, deliberately avoids questions of diffusion. Research funders like the National Institutes of Health reward elegant theory and rigorous study design above all. Questions about the potential for diffusion of the optimal treatment technologies are secondary at best.

By contrast, the goals of pharmaceutical companies are in many respects different from those of academic researchers. For pharmaceutical companies, it is neither necessary nor sufficient to extend the technological frontier—rather, the purpose of research is simply to produce agents that can be sold and used by customers. Policy changes in mental health have shifted the nature of the customer who is targeted by pharmaceutical companies.

In an era of centralized mental health decision-making authority, the pharmaceutical industry's customer was the mental health authority and the specialized physician. Research in several areas of medical care suggests that physicians give much greater weight to control of symptoms over freedom from side effects than patients do. In this climate, pharmaceutical companies would benefit from stressing research that focused on efficacy. By contrast, in an era of decentralized decision-making authority, producing products that can be readily prescribed by less specialized physicians and taken by less closely supervised consumers is likely to be a more successful strategy. The emphasis on consumer choice in mental health decision making is most evident with respect to antidepressants, which constitute the class of drug that is most frequently advertised directly to consumers (Rosenthal et al., 2002).

Research on the adoption of treatment technologies points to a further advantage of pharmaceutical companies in disseminating their products. The patent system gives a company exclusive property rights for eighteen years. This long protection period affords companies both an incentive to develop new products and the potential to enhance the performance of the product over time (Hall and Kahn, 2003). For example, a pharmaceutical company partners with epidemiologists to develop simple screens that physicians can use in diagnosing depression—which can then be treated with the pharmaceutical company's products.

Practitioner innovation is another important source of technological advance in many sectors. Many mental health providers are innovative in their practices. The return to such innovations, however, can rarely be appropriated by the innovator, which thereby reduces the incentive to disseminate information on the advance in practice. Furthermore, the costs of rigorously assessing the benefits of a new therapy or treatment strategy are usually too great to be borne by an individual provider. Instead, innovations initiated by providers usually enter the technological frontier only after they have undergone academic research.

This pattern has been particularly important in the development of new psychotherapies. Although considerable advances have been made in our understanding of the psychotherapies that can be effectively used to treat a variety of mental illnesses, there is little evidence that these new therapies are either easily delivered by the myriad mental health providers available or easily tolerated by mental health consumers (table 3.5).

There are several sources of exnovation. One is a market test whereby consumers reject one treatment in favor of another when the alternatives are equally effective. A second source of exnovation is based on a provider's greater understanding of evidence that a treatment is less safe and less effective than other reasonable alternatives. A third source of exnovation results from a technology's becoming inconsistent with the organization and financing of care. All three forces have been at work in mental health care.

Technological advances in mental health care over the past fifty years have

TABLE 3.5
Treatment Advances for Mental Disorders

	1955–1969	1970–1984	1985–2000
Schizophrenia	Neuroleptics (chlorpromazine, haloperidol)		Clozapine and other atypical antipsychotics (risperidone, olanzapine) for treatment-resistant schizophrenia Assertive Community Treatment
Depression	MAOIs (iproniazid, phenelzine) Tricyclic antidepressants (imipramine, amitriptyline) Interpersonal therapy Behavioral therapy	Cognitive therapy	SSRIs (fluoxetine, sertraline, paroxetine, fluvoxamine) CBT
Attention deficit hyperactivity disorder	Psychostimulants		
Anxiety disorders	Minor tranquilizers (meprobamate, benzodiazepines—diazepam, chlordiazepoxide) Imipramine for PD Desensitization therapy	High-potency benzodiazepines (alprazolam or Xanax) for panic disorder and generalized anxiety disorder (GAD) Exposure therapy Cognitive therapy	Tricyclic antidepressant clomipramine (Anafranil) for OCD SSRIs (for OCD, panic disorder, GAD, SAD, PTSD) CBT with exposure therapy
Bipolar disorder	Neuroleptics for mania and psychosis MAOIs and TCAs for depression Lithium (in Europe)	Lithium formally approved by FDA (1970)	Anticonvulsants for mood stabilization SSRIs ECT found efficacious Calcium channel blockers (verapamil) Atypical antipsychotics Psychosocial therapies

SOURCE: Data from Shorter, 1997; DiMasi and Lasagna, 2000; USFDA Orange Book, accessed 2003.

contributed significantly to the well-being of people with mental illness, but these gains are not primarily due to the greater efficacy of new treatments. Rather, since 1970 these improvements have come about primarily through advances that make it easier to diffuse treatment to more patients and providers.

CHAPTER 4

Health Care Financing
and Income Support

Between 1950 and 2000 the financing and delivery of mental health care underwent structural changes as dramatic as those in the Eastern European nations after the Soviet Union's disintegration. In a matter of twenty years, starting in the mid-1960s, mental health care moved largely from a centrally planned, state-owned and operated enterprise to a system dominated by market forces, though it still retained a large amount of public financing. These primary financing changes—not technological breakthroughs or demographic shifts—have transformed the lives of people with mental illness.

In the early 1960s choices about which services to provide and how much to spend on these services were made by state legislators. Legislators allocated a yearly budget for their state's centrally organized mental health system, whose focal point was the state mental hospital. People with a serious mental illness had few, if any, real choices about their care.

Today mentally ill individuals have become consumers, choosing their care—and allocating the financial resources associated with that care—from a broad array of institutions and services. They can usually weigh for themselves whether to enter a psychiatric hospital, a general hospital, a partial hospital (an institutional setting offering services similar to those of a hospital, without the overnight stay), a clinic, or a private office—each with its own assortment of services, providers, and intensities of care. Providers of care now compete for consumers on the basis of price, quality, and convenience—the very ingredients with which any business, whether a grocery store or an electronics outlet, vies for consumers. Health care markets differ from others, and the mental health care market has its own unique imperfections. Nonetheless, today there are markets for insurance and mental health care services where none existed before.[1]

The emergence of insurance and markets in mental health care turned individuals into consumers and thrust providers into the role of suppliers, with many of the commercial connotations of those labels. In the 1950s and early 1960s severely ill patients were cared for in what the sociologist Erving Goffman labeled "total institutions," which took pervasive control over all aspects of life. Outside institutional walls, less severely ill people sought counseling from a few public dispensaries or from office-based psychiatrists, for which they paid out of pocket. Today in the United States 86 percent of adults—and 80 percent of mentally ill adults—have some form of public or private insurance that confers varying degrees of protection against the high cost of care.[2]

Financing policies have been the principal driver of system change, as they have engineered the disintegration of the centralized mental health system. With its disintegration came the erosion of what we call mental health exceptionalism.

Financing Mental Health Care, 1950–2000

The first health economist to focus on mental health care financing was Rashi Fein. In *Economics of Mental Illness* (1958) he furnished an estimate of at least $1.14 billion for nominal spending in 1956. Fein estimated that state governments accounted for the lion's share of this funding. They were responsible for 59 percent of overall mental health care spending, while the federal government spent 25 percent. The remaining 16 percent came from other sources such as out-of-pocket payments and private insurance. Fein could not obtain data on private insurance. He did, however, estimate spending on private psychiatrists and private psychiatric hospitals on the basis of available information, and some of these costs may have been paid by private insurance.

Table 4.1 provides a summary of the level and composition of mental health service spending over the last five decades. Using data collected from a wide range of public and private sources, the table reports spending in current dollars. Spending grew more than seventyfold, from $1.14 billion in 1956 to $85.4 billion in 2001, faster than overall health care spending, with all the excess growth taking place in the 1956–71 period. Even after taking account of economy-wide inflation, mental health care spending grew dramatically over this period.

These changes occurred because of specific policy and market developments. First, Medicaid was established in 1965. Just six years later, in 1971, it already accounted for roughly 16 percent of all mental health spending. Medicaid contributed to a drastic reduction in states' share of direct spending on mental health services. In Fein's study states were responsible for 59 percent of overall spending in 1956. By 1971 the share of direct state spending dropped precipitously to about 23 percent, roughly the share today.

In fact, state spending share did not so much evaporate as shift. Since 1965 states have been required by federal law to make matching contributions to federal Medicaid spending. If states' Medicaid matching contributions are added to their direct outlays, total state spending was roughly 36 percent in 1971, 33 percent in 1987, 28 percent in 1997, and 35 percent in 2001. State funds shifted dramatically away from direct spending on services toward Medicaid matching.

The expansion of public and private insurance arrangements over the latter half of the century led to a marked decline in out-of-pocket spending, from nearly 36 percent in 1971 to about 13 percent in 2001. Millions of people who are not seriously mentally ill now have greater protection against financial losses associated with mental illness. Finally, the federal government's role in paying for mental health care has grown as a result of the 1965 passage of Medicaid and Medicare, two different forms of public health insurance. This, too, represented a shift in the form of funding, as the federal government began spending most of its mental health dollars through insurance mechanisms.

The changes in overall spending patterns are clear. Between 1956 and 1971 the state share of spending dropped by nearly half. Since 1971 there has been significant growth in the federal and private insurance shares, greater protection for consumers against financial losses, and stability in state spending.

The Delivery of Mental Health Services, 1950–2000

The locus and nature of mental health services delivered to patients also changed greatly in the postwar period. The magnitude of the shifts in care can be seen in data on treatment episodes: in 1955, 77 percent of treatment episodes took place in inpatient settings (state mental hospitals and other hospitals), whereas by 1975 only 28 percent were in inpatient facilities (U.S. President's Commission on Mental Health, 1978b, app. table 2). The absolute number of outpatient episodes is even more telling: the 379,000 outpatient treatment episodes in 1955 mushroomed thirteen years later to almost 2 million (Grob, 2001).

The shift away from state mental hospitals has been called *deinstitutionalization,* but the reality was that patients were often discharged to other types of institution—general hospitals or nursing homes—particularly after Medicaid was created in 1965. Indeed, instead of the term *deinstitutionalization,* many prefer to call the shift *transhospitalization* (Geller, 2000). Over the decade of the 1960s

TABLE 4.1
Level and Share of Spending for Mental Health Services, by Payer (in Current Dollars)

	1956	1971[a]	1987[b]	1997[b]	2001[c]
Medicare	—	2.6%	8.3%	12.8%	7.3%
Medicaid	—	14.2%	16.0%	20.4%	27.4%
Private insurance	—	12.3%	22.2%	23.9%	21.9%
Out of pocket	16.0%	35.6%	19.2%	16.9%	12.8%
State	59.0%	30.4%	25.3%	20.0%	23.4%
Other direct federal mental health spending[d]	25.0%	3.5%	6.1%	4.1%	5.0%
Miscellaneous	—	1.4%	2.9%	1.9%	2.2%
Total spending	$1.14 bn	$8.96 bn	$35.7 bn	$70.8 bn	$85.4 bn

[a] Levine and Levine (1975). To make the 1971 estimates comparable to the more recent estimates, we used estimates of the percentage of nursing home, hospital, and outpatient spending that was attributable to senile dementia, mental retardation, and related disorders not covered by the National Health Accounts approach. Using figures from Mark et al. (2005), we estimated that about 86% of nursing home spending was attributable to dementia. We allocated this spending according to aggregate shares by payers, largely Medicaid (60%), out-of-pocket spending (30%), and other payers. We then used data from US PCMH (1978b, app. table 10) to categorize the diagnostic mix by major types of treatment settings. We identified diagnoses that cover senile dementia and related conditions. These accounted for between 2% (outpatient) and 5% (state mental hospitals) of spending by setting. We subtracted these numbers from the total and allocated the amount subtracted to payer categories on the basis of the composition of spending in 1971.

[b] Coffey et al. (2000).

[c] Mark et al. (2005).

[d] These include expenditures such as the Veterans Administration and the Alcohol, Drug Abuse, and Mental Health block grant.

the nursing home population swelled from about 470,000 to almost 928,000, a nearly twofold growth (Grob, 2001).

The shift in care can be seen in table 4.2, which depicts trends from 1971 to 2001 in the composition of mental health services. The table highlights the diminished role of state mental hospitals, whose share of overall spending fell by more than two-thirds. At the same time, the use of general hospital psychiatric units grew as a portion of total spending on mental health care, from 9.7 percent in 1971 to 16 percent in 2001.

Reorienting the mental health system toward community-based treatment became the stated goal of national policy when President Kennedy created in 1963 the Community Mental Health Centers (CMHCs) program. Table 4.2 shows that by 1971 CMHCs and outpatient psychiatric clinics accounted for nearly 8 percent of specialty mental health spending. In terms of treatment episodes, CMHCs supplied 15.4 percent of all such episodes in the United States in 1971. That share rose to 24.7 percent by 1975 (U.S. President's Commission on Mental Health, 1978b, app. table 2).

The shift in emphasis away from public hospitals and toward community-

TABLE 4.2
Share of Spending for Specialty Mental Health Services

	1971[a]	1987[b]	1997[b]	2001[c]
State mental hospitals	23.0%	23.9%	13.3%	7.0%
Private psychiatric hospitals	3.0	7.0	7.2	14.0
General hospitals	9.7	16.6	16.3	16.0
Nursing homes	28.0	12.0	6.2	7.0
CMHCs/OP clinics	7.9	10.6	15.1	18.0
Psychiatrists	8.7	7.7	9.7	8.7
Psychologists/social worker	1.0	10.3	13.4	8.0
Drugs	5.6	7.5	12.3	21.0

NOTE: Percentages do not add to 100 because some services are not shown.
[a] Levine and Levine (1975).
[b] Coffey et al. (2000).
[c] State and private psychiatric estimates are based on Mark et al. (2005) and expenditure shares from U.S. DHHS CMHS, 2004, table 8a.

based treatment was accompanied by growth in the mental health professions, especially psychotherapists. Markets for psychotherapy have grown quickly since the 1960s, and table 4.2 shows astonishing growth (thirteenfold) in the share of treatment resources spent on psychologists and social workers. The share of spending on psychotherapy appears to have declined between 1997 and 2001.

Innovations in pharmacology, along with expanded insurance coverage for prescription drugs, propelled spending on drugs. The spending share for drugs grew from about 5.6 percent in 1971 to 12.3 percent in 1997. The growth was even more rapid from 1987 to 2001, a time of substantial innovation in psychopharmacology, when the annual growth rate in spending on prescription drugs ranged from about 9 to 22 percent (Coffey et al., 2000; Mark et al., 2005).

To some extent, the shift in the pattern of care toward community-based services reflects changing attitudes and beliefs. The immediate post–World War II period ushered in a period of optimism about the potential for community-based treatment (Grob, 1994, 2001). During the war the military had successfully pioneered treatment of soldiers' stress disorders near their base, rather than transporting them back to military hospitals. Many military psychiatrists, once they returned to civilian life, tried to adapt these techniques of bringing care closer to home. They were also influenced by the Freudian emphasis on social and environmental factors in shaping mental health. Some hoped that early intervention in the community would prevent hospitalization.

This positive vision of the benefits of community-based treatment occurred in parallel with growing concern about the benefits and costs of institutional care.

Reports about the quality of care in mental hospitals outraged the public, particularly in a climate that placed growing importance on respecting the rights of psychiatric patients. But the shift in care owes much more to the profound changes in the financing of care over this period than to these changing perceptions.

The Changing Price of Mental Health Care

The basic institutions that govern the financing of health care in the United States today were developed between 1955 and 1975. Private employer-sponsored health insurance grew rapidly, public health insurance for elderly persons and segments of the poor and disabled populations was enacted, and social insurance[3] for elderly and disabled persons was expanded. These new health and social welfare programs profoundly affected the financing and delivery of mental health care.

Within the mental health sector, beginning in the 1950s, an attack was mounted on the public mental hospital, the dominant institution for psychiatric care (Grob, 2001). In the wake of highly publicized revelations about deplorable conditions in public mental hospitals, a central element of the attack was a set of legal challenges to protect the rights of patients to receive active treatment. The legal challenges established quality-of-care standards requiring many state hospitals to restructure the "production" process to deliver higher-quality services (Rubin, 1978, 1980).

The institutional changes in the financing of health care more generally, together with these transformations in the mental health system, brought about major changes in how much households, private insurers, and local, state, and federal governments had to pay for mental health care—that is, the "price" of mental health care. This price is determined by the division of financial responsibility assigned to these parties (by legislation or contract) and, as is true in other contexts, affects economic choices and the resulting burden of expenditure.[4]

Medicaid and Medicare

The 1965 enactment of Medicare and Medicaid legislation had even more profound effects on mental health care delivery. Spearheaded by President Lyndon Johnson, Medicaid and Medicare newly amended different parts of the Social Security Act. With the reduction of poverty his intention, Johnson saw these programs as "pillars of protection upon which all our people can safely build their lives and their hopes" (quoted in Min DeParle, 2000).

Medicaid established a form of public health insurance for segments of the poor and disabled populations where none had existed previously. Those eligible for

Medicaid included certain poor children and their mothers, disabled people (and, after 1972, those eligible for SSI), and certain Medicare beneficiaries (US HCFA, 2000). In practice, Medicaid established a voucherlike mechanism that allowed beneficiaries to purchase mental health care from any provider willing to accept Medicaid fees as payment in full. Poor and disabled Medicaid enrollees with mental disorders were, for the first time, able to choose among general hospital psychiatric units, community mental health centers, outpatient mental health clinics, and, to a more limited extent, office-based psychiatrists and psychologists.

The enactment of Medicaid also caused enormous changes in the price of mental health services to state governments. This occurred in several ways. Medicaid is financed by a matching grant from the federal government to each state. A state's matching obligation is by law inversely related to its per capita income, but the state's obligation cannot exceed 50 percent.[5] Under this formula, the price of mental health care to any state ranges between 20 and 50 percent of overall Medicaid costs. Correspondingly, the price to the federal government ranges from 50 percent to a high of about 80 percent. Medicaid, in short, substantially reduced the price of mental health care to the states.

Specialty mental hospitals (including state mental hospitals and private psychiatric hospitals) were explicitly excluded from Medicaid payment under the Institution of Mental Disease (IMD) exclusion (US HCFA, 1992). The IMD exclusion was based on 1950 amendments to the Social Security Act that precluded cash assistance payments for patients in IMDs and for medical patients with a diagnosis of psychosis. The reasons behind the IMD exclusion were both economic and humanitarian. First, Congress wanted to prevent cost shifting from state budgets onto the federal budget. "Responsibility for the treatment of persons in mental hospitals . . . is that of the MH agency of the State" (US HR, 1965). Second, Congress wanted to encourage elderly people with mental disorders to be treated in less restrictive settings than specialty mental hospitals (US HCFA, 1992).[6]

One major effect of Medicaid and its IMD exclusion was to prompt states to shift care from state mental hospitals to nursing homes. Economics was paramount, for the states knew that costs would be largely assumed by the federal government. The daily spending for an inpatient in a public mental hospital in 1971 was about thirty dollars. The daily spending on nursing home care was lower, and, under Medicaid, a state paid only 20 to 50 percent of the cost. So states saved a large amount of money by discharging patients from mental hospitals to nursing homes. Similarly, as long as the daily costs were less than double those of state hospitals, states had a strong incentive to shift the setting of care to general hospital psychiatric units.

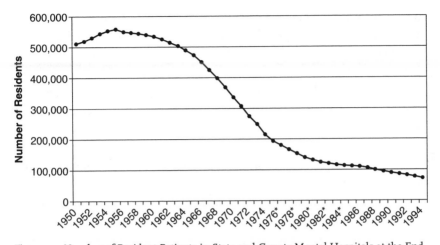

Figure 4.1. Number of Resident Patients in State and County Mental Hospitals at the End of the Year, 1950–1994. Asterisk indicates linear interpolation.
SOURCE: Data from Manderscheid et al., 2001.

Figure 4.1 shows the trend in the resident census of state and county mental hospitals. After peaking in 1955, the resident census of patients began to fall at a modest rate (1.5% per year) over the next ten years. But in the years following 1965 the rate of decline was about 8 percent. The decline was even more pronounced for the elderly. People aged sixty-five years and older had large reductions in use of state hospitals. Between 1955 and 1973 there was a 70.6 percent reduction in the rate of such hospitalizations among the elderly, while the rate of nursing home use grew substantially. In 1960, 262 of every 100,000 elderly persons were residents of nursing homes, compared to 456 per 100,000 in 1970, a 74 percent increase (Kramer, 1977).

The changing pattern of nursing home use for elderly people with mental disorders clearly reflected the changing price to states after Medicaid's creation. In 1963, two years before Medicaid, nursing homes accounted for roughly 53 percent of all institutional care for elderly people with mental disorders. By 1969, four years after Medicaid, nursing homes accounted for nearly 75 percent of institutional care for elderly people with mental disorders (ibid., app. table 7). The 1977 National Nursing Home Survey reported that about 87 percent of nursing home residents had a diagnosis of senility or a major psychiatric disorder (US DHEW, 1980). For the vast majority, psychiatric disorders were recorded as a secondary diagnosis to prevent a nursing home's being classified as an IMD. If 50 percent or more of a nursing home's residents (regardless of age) have a primary (as opposed to a secondary) psychiatric diagnosis, the nursing home is classified as an IMD (Shadish et al., 1989). If so classified, a nursing home would lose all its Medicaid funding.

Medicare, enacted in 1965, provides health insurance to elderly and some disabled people. All Americans age sixty-five and older are eligible for Part A of Medicare, which pays for hospital care. Enrollment in Part B, which pays for professional and other services, is optional and thus requires a premium be paid. Nearly all Part A beneficiaries enroll in Part B.

Medicare's Part A coverage is generous with respect to inpatient psychiatric care when compared to typical private insurance. There are no limits on covered days, except for freestanding psychiatric hospitals, where inpatient care is limited to 190 days over the course of a lifetime. Between 1965 and 1990 Medicare's coverage for outpatient mental health care was more restrictive than coverage for other types of outpatient health care. Medicare law required beneficiaries to pay 50 percent of the cost of outpatient mental health treatment, rather than the 20 percent required for other health services. By law, beneficiaries also faced a limit of five hundred dollars in allowable charges in a year (which did not apply to other types of care), and the only eligible providers were physicians. From the mid-1980s to 1990, in a bid to improve benefits, reduce discrimination, and bring mental health coverage in line with other health coverage, Congress enacted four legislative changes to Medicare that relaxed the spending limit placed on outpatient psychiatric care, covered medical management visits at the same level as all other outpatient medical visits, added psychologists and social workers as covered providers, and included partial hospitalization as a covered service (Lave and Goldman, 1990; Rosenbach and Ammering, 1997).

Medicare's effect in the decades after its introduction was to substantially expand inpatient mental health care coverage for elderly patients in private hospitals. From 1987 to 1992 the legislative changes led to a doubling in overall per capita spending on mental health services. Access dramatically rose too, with a 73 percent climb in the number of new users (Frank et al., 1999). These expansions created insurance revenues for services that had previously been largely funded by out-of-pocket payments or through direct grants from state governments to community-based providers.

Private Insurance

Modern employer-sponsored health insurance began to take hold during World War II, and its growth thereafter was driven by federal policy and union activity (Somers and Somers, 1961; Starr, 1982). A ruling by the Labor Control Board in 1943 stated that employer contributions to health insurance and pensions did not count as wages. Given the existence of price and wage controls, health insurance became a mechanism by which employers could compete for scarce labor during the war years. The number of people with health insurance tripled. Then, in the immediate postwar years, health benefits became a focal point for labor negotiations. By 1958 about 68 percent of the population had private health insurance of some type. About 75 percent of that insurance was employer-sponsored (Somers and Somers, 1961).

By the late 1960s the vast majority of employer-sponsored health plans, 92 percent, offered some coverage for inpatient and outpatient mental health care (Reed, 1975). Typical coverage among private plans carried special restrictions not found for other types of care: relatively high levels of cost sharing (i.e., higher co-payments), special limits on utilization, and dollar caps on overall coverage. The most common features applying to mental health care coverage were 20 percent copayment rates for inpatient care, 50 percent copayment rates for outpatient care, a thirty-day limit on covered inpatient care, a twenty-five-visit limit on outpatient visits, and caps of two thousand dollars or less on total annual spending.[7] In addition, most health plans excluded coverage for care in either private psychiatric hospitals or publicly owned mental hospitals (ibid.).

This benefit package did not provide protection against large financial losses, which is arguably the most valuable reason for insurance (Arrow, 1963). Instead, mental health insurance offered some coverage for the most affordable financial losses and virtually no protection against large and potentially ruinous expenses for treatment of mental disorders.

Special limitations on mental health coverage arose for several reasons. All of them apply to health coverage in general, but even more strongly to mental health coverage in particular. The first is an economic phenomenon called *moral hazard.* Higher levels of cost sharing for mental health coverage than for other health coverage are justified by insurers because the demand for mental health services is more responsive to the terms of coverage, especially under traditional indemnity (fee-for-service) insurance (Newhouse et al., 1993; Frank and McGuire, 2000). Lowering co-payments induced much greater additional use of outpatient mental health care than similar reductions induced in other areas of medical spending. The second reason for special limits stems from competition between health plans to avoid high-cost enrollees. Because people who expect to have extensive need for treatment tend to choose health plans with more generous coverage, plans offering deep coverage for mental health care tend to attract a disproportionately high number of costly cases (relative to other types of illnesses). Those costly cases place the plan at a competitive disadvantage when compared to other plans in a way unrelated to the plan's efficiency or quality. This economic phenomenon is known as *adverse selection*. Adverse selection creates incentives for plans to limit certain types of coverage so as to avoid attracting "bad risks." The problem of adverse selection led to a market failure in private mental health care coverage: the private market failed to meet a societal goal.

This market failure was exacerbated by the existence of the large public mental health system, which had historically taken responsibility for serving people with severe and persistent mental disorders and thus essentially furnished protection against catastrophic costs. Private-sector coverage was, in effect, crowded out by the existence of the public mental health system. The confluence of these forces—moral hazard, adverse selection, and the presence of a large public mental health system— led to relatively limited private insurance coverage for mental health care.

Crafting responses to perceived market failures in insurance coverage for mental health care has been a persistent role of mental health policy since the 1960s. In 1977 the President's Commission on Mental Health debated how to address market failures. The report summarized the discussion as follows: "The panel considered various ways of enlarging the financing of mental health services in non-Federal programs. These included technical assistance, persuasion, and other forms of encouragement. . . . They also discussed urging or requiring states to mandate enlarged mental health coverage. The panel did not agree on preferences among these options" (US PCMH, 1978b, 514).

State governments regulate private insurance markets. They began to address market failures in insurance for mental health care in the early 1970s. Connecticut passed the nation's first mandated mental health coverage law in 1971 (Frank, 1989b). It established minimum levels of coverage for all private insurance sold in the state. Over the subsequent decade, about eighteen states followed Connecticut's lead. State laws served both the public interest and government's self-interest. The states' public interest was to limit the consequences of adverse selection. The states' self-interest was to shift costs for some mental health services from their budgets to private insurance plans. McGuire and Montgomery (1982) showed that expanded private insurance arising from mandated health insurance did indeed reduce states' financial obligations to community mental health centers. Frank (1985) estimated that states passing mandates spent less on public inpatient mental health care than did otherwise similar states.

Laws that mandated the provision of mental health benefits did not generally require that these benefits be provided on the same terms as general health benefits. Beginning in the 1990s, and taking up a call that had first been sounded by President Kennedy, advocates argued for parity—or equality—of benefits for general and mental health care. During the 1990s several states began to require some parity in mental health benefits, usually by eliminating hospital day or visit restrictions. Then, in 1996, Congress passed a parity act, which required elimination of yearly and lifetime dollar caps on mental health coverage.

Legal Requirements to Improve State Hospital Care

Changes in the price of mental health care also came about through legal challenges. During the 1970s a number of court decisions established that psychiatric patients treated in state mental hospitals have a right to treatment. In the case of *Wyatt v. Stickney* (503 F. 2d 1305 [5th Cir., 1974]), Judge Frank Johnson wrote out a detailed set of standards regarding what constituted a minimally acceptable quality of care in public psychiatric hospitals. The standards defined adequate staffing, specified a humane physical and psychological environment, and required individual treatment plans. Meanwhile, public outrage mounted over reports of inhumane conditions. Both the political environment and judicial decisions pressured states to invest more in state mental hospitals' physical plants and staffing levels. These investments raised the costs of care. For example, meeting the staffing standard of *Wyatt* alone was expected to raise the average state's costs by 6 percent (Rubin, 1980). Spending increases tied to judicial decisions amounted to about $404 million in 1977, or 15 percent of mental health spending. The effect of sharp price hikes due to new regulations was to lower demand for state mental health services. Later estimates suggested that state governments were quite sensitive to the price of state hospital services, which bolstered the view that judicial regulation contributed to the reduced use of public mental hospitals (Frank, 1985).

Community Mental Health Centers

Many of the price changes that shifted care toward the community were unintended. By contrast, the Community Mental Health Centers (CMHCs) program, championed by President Kennedy and authorized by Congress in 1963, had the direct intention of reducing the price of community-based mental health services to people with mental health problems and thereby encourage access to care.

The CMHC program was the first direct federal commitment to mental health care in more than one hundred years (Sharfstein, 2000). It consisted primarily of construction grants for communities to build outpatient centers, to which it then gave operating funds for the first few years. Designed as seed money, funding in the early years was supposed to attract, and eventually be replaced by, third-party payments. Because of the federal budget constraints created by the Vietnam War, however, the CMHCs' operating budgets did not rise to expected levels. Further compounding the problem was the fact that in 1968 Congress passed legislation expanding the role of CMHCs to serve new groups—substance abusers, children, and older people. With a broadened mission and fewer than expected resources, CMHCs seldom accorded priority to severely mentally ill people (US GAO, 1977; Grob, 2001). That is, with a limited fixed budget and responsibility for serving a local population, CMHCs chose to serve a great number of less impaired and lower-cost people rather than disproportionately allocating their budget to high-cost severely ill people. A Government Accounting Office report— *Returning the Mentally Disabled to the Community: Government Needs to Do More* (GAO, 1977)—highlighted the failure of CMHCs as an organization to serve people with severe mental disorders.

The design of CMHC funding—financing capacity building rather than operations—meant that it also had relatively smaller effects on the price of community-based care than did the large financing programs that followed. Indeed, an event study analysis by Gronfein (1985) found that the CMHC program was vastly overshadowed by Medicaid in terms of its influence on the rate of decline of number of patients treated in public mental hospitals. His estimates indicate that Medicaid's effect was about four times more significant than the CMHCs' in reducing the population of public mental hospitals.

OBRA 90 and the Block Grant Program

The Reagan administration, within its first months of office in 1981, ushered in a reversal of federal policy. The federal government gave back to the states most of the direct responsibility for mental health care that it had only recently assumed. The process unfolded when President Reagan proposed to rescind the Mental Health Systems Act of 1980. That act had redefined the role of CMHCs and given them a special emphasis on services for the most vulnerable population groups. Under the president's prodding, Congress repealed the act less than a year after the departing Carter administration had passed it. Through separate legislation, the Omnibus Budget Reconciliation Act of 1981 (U.S. Congress, 1981), Congress bundled together the funding for CMHCs and other so-called categorical federal mental health programs. The combination of categorical programs was converted into a block grant, a lump sum to every state with few strings attached. Congress also cut overall funding significantly (Jacobson et al., 1996).

The block grant was initially designed to give states the flexibility to design their own mental health programs. It was intended to improve the efficiency of federal spending and make it more responsive to local conditions. It aimed to create incentives for state and local government to devote money to activities with the largest local payoff rather than activities defined by national federal program rules.

In practice, however, the intended flexibility of mental health care financing under the block grant turned out to be short-lived (ibid.). Spending priorities, program development guidelines, and reporting requirements multiplied rapidly during the late 1980s and early 1990s. The main structural effect of the block grant seems to have been a cut in federal spending levels that took place in the early 1980s.

Supporting Life in the Community

Changes in the price of mental health services led to upheavals in the nature and sites of mental health care, particularly for people with serious mental illness. Moving people with serious illnesses into the community, however, meant giving up both institutionally based mental health care and the array of other services—food, housing, clothing—that had also been the responsibility of the total institution. Policy makers designed coherent aftercare models to provide these services, but ultimately the largest contributor to community support came through unrelated federal legislation that provided stable cash support and housing to disabled people.

Income Support

Two new federal income-support programs were introduced in the 1960s and 1970s: Supplemental Security Income (SSI) and Social Security Disability Income (SSDI). These programs gave cash support to people with a disability, including a psychiatric disability.[8] Their creation added more resources to support people with severe mental illnesses and produced greater diversity and complexity in funding streams.

Enacted in 1972, the federal SSI program replaced a patchwork of state programs that had provided more limited assistance to disabled and aged persons. SSI began paying benefits in 1974. It was designed as a means-tested program providing payments to low-income, disabled adults and children, regardless of work history. Disability was defined as a condition that prevents one from engaging in substantial gainful activity. Although the federal SSI payment level was set nationally, a number of states supplement federal SSI payments. SSI recipients living in poor households are also eligible for food stamps and, in most states, for Medicaid.

Children are also eligible for SSI, and children with mental disorders have been a focus of policy attention in the program. In 1990 new rules promulgated by the Social Security Administration expanded the number of SSI-qualifying conditions to include attention deficit hyperactivity disorder (ADHD) and other mental disorders in children. Around the same time the Supreme Court in *Zebley v. Sullivan* (493 U.S. 521 [1990]) ruled that the SSI definition of disability be expanded to include global impairment independent of specific mental disorder. The net result of these rulings was to increase the number of children with ADHD and other mental disorders on SSI by 66 percent from 1990 to 1992 alone. Between 1989 and 1996 the total number of children receiving SSI almost quadrupled, from 275,000 to 1,000,000.

After 1996 the tide reversed. Intense federal pressures to decrease the budget deficit, combined with extensive negative publicity about fraud in the system, prompted Congress to tighten eligibility and impairment criteria and require reassessment of many children on SSI, beginning with those qualified through a diagnosis of ADHD. In the end more than 100,000 children, most with mental disorders, lost SSI and SSI-related Medicaid eligibility.

Social Security Disability Insurance (SSDI) was enacted in 1956 but it was not until several years later that the program became a significant source of financial support for people with mental illness. SSDI had initially been restricted to people fifty years old and older. Then, in 1960, the program began to pay benefits to those becoming disabled after they qualified for social security by working for at least ten years.[9] The level of benefits depend on past earnings, so people with higher pre-disability earnings receive greater payments than do those with low earnings. SSI supplements SSDI payments for low-income disabled people. People who become disabled and qualify for SSDI can receive Medicare after two years.

Participation in SSDI grew through 1980. For example, from 1970 to 1975 the number of SSDI disabled-worker beneficiaries increased by 45 percent (figures cited in Goldman and Gattozzi, 1988). Then, as part of an effort to reduce federal spending under President Carter, Congress passed the 1980 disability amendments to the Social Security Act. The amendments required a disability review at least once every three years for persons not determined to be permanently disabled. In 1982 the Reagan administration began to require reviews to be conducted in person in SSA offices, and it applied very stringent criteria to the reviews. The consequence of these reviews, which began in 1983, was that some 500,000 people lost eligibility for these programs. Goldman and Gattozzi estimated that "one-fourth of 130,500 beneficiaries dropped from the rolls during the first full year of the reviews were mentally impaired," even though they constituted fewer than 10 percent of beneficiaries. There was no mental health exceptionalism in these reviews—people with mental illness were not expressly singled out. That, however, was the unintended consequence. Among the disabled, people with mental illnesses are disproportionately young and able-bodied because onset often occurs in the late teens and twenties. Lack of attention to the unique features of mental illness meant that people with mental illness disproportionately lost their benefits (ibid.).

In response to the high disenrollment rate, Congress passed the 1984 Disability Benefits Reform Act, which specified that benefits could be terminated only if a person had experienced medical improvements in his or her condition and was now capable of sustained gainful activity.

Participation in the SSI and SSDI program has been increasing rapidly over the past decade. Since the late 1980s SSI eligibility as a result of mental disorders has been one of the fastest-growing components of the program (Stapleton et al., 1998). In 1996 Congress eliminated eligibility for SSI and SSDI for people whose primary disabling condition was drug abuse or alcohol addiction. About 60 percent of this group lost their eligibility for the program. But the effect was somewhat blunted, for many with substance use disorders continued to be eligible by virtue of a co-occurring mental disorder: about 43 percent of these people have at least one mental disorder (Kessler et al., 1994).

Housing

As we will show in chapter 7, SSI and SSDI have become mainstays of life for people with severe mental illness. Yet income support provided by these programs is often insufficient to pay the costs of housing. Thus, direct federal housing support is also extremely important to people with severe illness. Research during the 1980s and 1990s showed that people with severe and persistent mental illness who live in stable, high-quality housing in neighborhoods with newer housing stock have better clinical outcomes and use fewer health and mental health services than do severely mentally ill people in low-quality living arrangements (Newman et al., 1994; Harkness et al., 2004).

In 1970 the federal government began to subsidize rental housing for low-income tenants through the Section 8 certificate and voucher program. The vouchers and certificates give recipients a subsidy set at the fair-market rent, which is the 40th percentile of the local rental market for standard-quality units. About 13 percent of those served by the program today are disabled.

In addition to Section 8, several federal initiatives have also had the goal of providing supported housing to people with disabilities. These include the 1978

Community Support Program demonstration project for people with serious mental illness and various programs authorized under the 1987 McKinney Act, including the Shelter Plus Care program and the Supportive Housing Program. The McKinney Act provides block grants to state and local governments to develop supported housing for people at risk of homelessness.

Levels of funding authorization for housing assistance programs have fluctuated substantially over time. Between 1978 and 1989 funding for housing programs declined dramatically. Funding authorization increased markedly between 1991 and 1994 but has dropped again since then.

Together, federal income and housing support programs indirectly reduced the price to states of supplying mental health care in the community rather than in institutions. By substituting for the life necessities component of institutional care, they enabled people with mental illness to make use of community-based treatment services.

Assessing the Effects of Institutional Change

As our review suggests, an array of major policy changes altered the prices of mental health care to various payers in different settings. To assess the quantitative impact of these changes on the financing and locus of care, we conducted an event study for the period 1950–99 (Summarized in figure 4.2). We examined the effect of these major policy changes on direct spending (per capita) on mental health by states—an indicator of financing changes—and on the resident population (per capita) of state mental hospitals—an indicator of changes in the locus of care.

We collected states' historical spending patterns from the Census of State Government. We used data from a category of expenditures that included mental hospitals and direct mental health services, as well as some other health programs. We obtained data on state hospital censuses from a series of National Institute

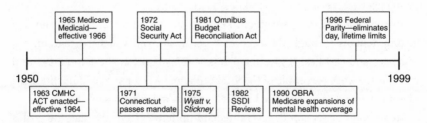

Figure 4.2. Mental Health Financing Time Line

TABLE 4.3
Regression Results: State Spending and State Hospital Residents per Capita

Event/variable	Natural Log of Spending/Population, 1950–1999 Newey[a]	Residents/Population, 1950–1999 OLS[b]	Residents/Population, 1950–1999 Newey[a]
Medicaid/Medicare	0.093*	−0.233*	−0.233
	(2.17)	(2.19)	(1.43)
CMHC	−0.008	−0.149	−0.149
	(0.81)	(1.66)	(1.66)
Wyatt v. Stickney	0.089	−0.05	−0.05
	(1.58)	(0.34)	(0.25)
Block grant	−0.088**	0.078	0.078
	(3.85)	(0.88)	(1.02)
SSI/DI changes	0.021	0.240*	0.240*
	(0.86)	(3.11)	(2.151)
SSI (1972)	0.078**	−0.392*	−0.392**
	(2.86)	(2.86)	(3.11)
OBRA 90	0.053**	0.160	0.160
	(3.11)	(1.67)	(1.62)
Mandates	0.018**	−0.023	−0.003
	(2.89)	(0.33)	(0.13)
Time	0.087*	−0.204**	−0.204
	(2.13)	(2.77)	(1.37)
Time^2	−0.001*	0.001	0.001
	(2.23)	(1.80)	(0.96)
ln population	−2.27	7.184	7.184
	(1.41)	(1.89)	(0.98)
Constant	31.85	−81.79	−81.79
	(1.28)	(1.81)	(0.94)
F statistic		F=696	
	22,811	R^2=0.99	42,403

NOTE: t statistics are in parentheses.
[a] Estimates are based on Newey adjusted standard errors for auto-correlated errors maximum lag 15.
[b] Ordinary least-squares estimator
*$p<0.05$
**$p<0.01$

of Mental Health (Kramer, 1977) and Substance Abuse and Mental Health Services Administration reports (U.S. DHHS CMHS, 2001b and prior years). The key events we identified in the history of mental health financing are displayed on the time line. We obtained the effective dates for these events from legislative histories, spending records, and government statistics.[10]

Table 4.3 presents results from regression analyses for the two outcomes: direct state mental health care spending per capita and state hospital residents per capita. State direct mental health care spending has grown throughout the period. Both the creation of Medicaid and the establishment of the modern SSI program resulted in significantly higher rates of state mental health care spending and lower rates of use of state mental hospitals. As our discussion above suggested, these policies reduced the price of mental health services in the community. (SSI provided income support in the community.) Medicaid, through the federal match, offered states community-based care at a discount. States have shifted the design of public mental health services in order to capture federal matching dollars. One element of this strategy has been to use state direct spending as state match contributions for Medicaid. Thus, the positive and significant coefficients for both SSI and Medicare-Medicare events suggest that though on-budget spending increased, those dollars were increasingly tied to Medicaid policy in terms of allocation choices (see Frank, Goldman, and Hogan, 2003, for an elaboration of this point). The Medicaid and SSI effect on the rate of state hospital use is consistently negative and statistically significant. Although the net effects of these programs on state mental health care spending were positive, the enactment of Medicaid and the creation of SSI shifted the emphasis in mental health care away from public mental hospital settings. Similarly, we find, as did Gronfein (1985), that the CMHC program served to reduce the populations of state mental hospitals, but that the estimated effect was considerably smaller than the effect of Medicaid, and CMHCs did not affect total state spending.

Increasing numbers of mandates for mental health benefits in private health insurance had a negative and significant effect on levels of state spending for mental health, but no clear effect on state hospital use. This pattern is consistent with a substitution of private insurance funding only for public funding of outpatient care. People with private insurance are less likely to have been users of public institutions. The estimated coefficient indicates that each additional mandated benefit statute reduces a state's mental health spending by about 1.8 percent. We did not find that the *Wyatt* decision, OBRA 90, which expanded mental health coverage under Medicare, or the 1981 block grant had any significant effect on state hospital use patterns.

Financing Changes in the 1990s: Managed Care

The rising cost of health care, and particularly of mental health care, throughout this period led to cost-containment efforts. In the 1990s managed care became the preeminent cost-containment strategy, replacing traditional indemnity insurance as the dominant way to organize and finance health care in the United States. Managed care began in the private sector, but it eventually spread to the public sector, particularly Medicaid.

The distinctive features of mental health service provision led to a design for managed care in mental health that was somewhat different from that for health care more generally. The most striking development has been the managed behavioral health care "carve-out." Traditionally, a health care purchaser (e.g., a major corporation) contracted with a single insurance plan to cover a full range of health risks. In the managed care era, purchasers began to offer beneficiaries an opportunity to make a choice among many health plans. Some purchasers also began to "carve out" certain benefits, meaning that they separated the health insurance function by disease or class of service and then contracted separately for the management of each (Frank et al., 1995). In this situation, carving out mental health benefits eliminates the possibility that adverse selection by people with mental health needs will lead to a reduction in a plan's mental health benefits.

General health plans may also choose to carve out mental health care to mental health specialty vendors. Integrated managed care plans are likely to be motivated by economies of specialization. In particular, specialty managed behavioral health care organizations offer specialized networks of providers that cannot be efficiently organized by many integrated health plans. They also possess expertise in mental health care and substance abuse care and their management.

Managed behavioral health care, introduced first in the private market and later in Medicaid, has had powerful effects on treatment patterns and spending for mental health services. Behavioral plans have achieved savings by reducing the number of days of inpatient care for mental and addictive disorders, reducing the prices paid to providers, and limiting the numbers of visits per outpatient treatment episode. Estimated reductions in mental health spending for both Medicaid programs and private insurance plans have ranged from about 15 to 45 percent (Sturm, 1999; Frank and Lave, 2003).

Perhaps surprisingly, managed behavioral health care has also been associated with higher rates of access to care and reduced cost-sharing requirements for enrollees. Shifting from high cost sharing to use management has reduced the up-front cost of initiating care. Managed care's quest to save money has generated concerns about lowered quality of care, but studies to date have not consistently shown evidence of quality reductions (or improvements). There is, however, some evidence that people with schizophrenia fare less well than do other Medicaid beneficiaries enrolled in managed care (Chang et al., 1998; Manning et al., 1999).

Managed care has had a particularly profound effect on weakening the role of many state mental health systems, exacerbating the institutional effects of the introduction of Medicaid. States increasingly rely on private managed behavioral health care companies to manage Medicaid mental health care. They also transform other sources of publicly funded services into Medicaid-eligible services and populations, whose management then shifts to private managed behavioral care companies. In combination, these effects have privatized much of the management of public mental health care.

The rise of managed behavioral health care may also limit the state's regulatory power in the private sector. Managed behavioral health care companies control costs without using the formal benefit design and cost-sharing limits that have been the subject of state-mandated benefit laws. The ability of states to regulate the private sector and address insurance market failures through these statutes may thus be weakened in the presence of managed behavioral health care (Frank et al., 2001).

Conclusions

Since 1950 the main policies affecting mental health care have had three primary direct effects. They have created insurance mechanisms to replace public financing and provision; they have altered the prices of deploying specific types of treatment resources (especially public mental hospitals); and they have used decentralized markets for insurance and treatment services to allocate resources in mental health care.

These policies have pumped significantly more resources into the mental health system. They have created enormous incentives for states to move the mental health delivery system away from specialized institutions and toward community-based treatment, a development further spurred by the adoption of managed care. Regulation of private insurance markets has improved the efficiency of private-sector coverage.

Together, these policies—Medicaid and Medicare, SSI and SSDI, increased reliance on insurance mechanisms for financing mental health care—have steered the provision of mental health services into the mainstream of U.S. health care delivery. Thus, over the past fifty years the United States has transformed mental health delivery from a centralized planned activity run by the states to a pluralistic, market-oriented system of care. The consequence has been to exchange a set of bureaucratic failures and tight budgets that took responsibility for all care for a circumscribed population for a vastly richer, decentralized system of care that suffers from market failure and allows some people with significant impairments to fall through the cracks.

CHAPTER 5

The Supply of Mental Health Services

Public and private spending on mental health services and social services that improve the well-being of people with mental illness have expanded tremendously since 1950. An infusion of new funding, coupled with the renewed professional optimism about the potential of mental health treatment that, in part, prompted that funding, spurred a vast expansion of institutional and professional mental health supply. This expansion in supply, in turn, led to greater use of services and lower unit prices for those services, and these developments were beneficial to people with mental illness. In addition, several aspects of the expansion in supply were both peculiar to mental health care and had notable effects on well-being.

One distinctive feature has been the role of policy outside the mental health sectors in affecting the supply of services. Changes in institutional and professional capacity have been quite responsive to changes in the expected financial returns from training for a career in this sector, rather than another. Here, too, the mainstream has exerted its force; public policy affecting the return to *alternative* career investments and treatment capacity outlays has often been as important as any mental health-specific policy in altering the supply of services. People with mental illnesses, as well as those who finance their care, have been the unanticipated beneficiaries of policies aimed at controlling other aspects of health care costs.

The nature of the supply expansion in mental health care was unique. The expansion consisted of not only an increase in the number of mental health providers, but also a substantial extension of the definition of what constitutes a mental health care provider. In 1950 the term, when applied to professionals, referred almost exclusively to physicians trained as psychiatrists. Today a wide array of expert providers—from counselors to social workers to psychologists to subspecialty psychiatrists—serve people with mental illness, and the vast majority of such specialty providers are not physicians at all. Moreover, in recent years primary care doctors have become increasingly involved in the treatment of mental health problems in their patients. This enlarging of the set of mental health care providers has given people with mental illness unprecedented choices. At the same time, because the lines of demarcation among these professionals are often fuzzy, both public and private purchasers have benefited from competition within and among provider groups.

A similar pattern occurred on the institutional side. The provision of inpatient mental health services, once the nearly exclusive province of large public inpatient facilities, became a role shared among the few remaining public facilities, a fluctuating number of private for-profit psychiatric hospitals, and a growing number of general hospital psychiatric units. Except in the case of forensic (i.e., criminal or corrections-involved) patients, it is increasingly difficult to draw sharp distinctions between the populations now served in these varied facilities.

A third feature has been the close linkage between mental health suppliers and public policy makers. For all their diversity, mental health professionals share a dependence on public and publicly regulated financing streams and a historic link between public mental hospitals and the medical profession. These strong ties to governmental agencies and to a history of dealing with regulation of professional practices have made mental health professionals unusually adept at securing public benefits. New professional groups have pursued and generally achieved licensure at the state level. They have succeeded in persuading state legislatures to require private insurers to compensate them for their services. They have lobbied, often effectively, to maintain institutions that provide them with staff positions. By capturing regulatory interest and power, mental health professionals were for many years able to maintain economic returns above competitive levels.

The ability of professionals to manipulate the political process, or regulatory capture, exacerbate the inherent difficulties of managing a system with a diverse range of patients and providers. As new provider alternatives arise, regulators and purchasers must determine how to set payments and utilization-control policies that optimally allocate resources. In the case of mental health services, differences in the severity of illness have always complicated these financing decisions, as was illustrated by our discussion of CMHCs in chapter 4. The growing array of institutional and professional providers—including the development of new treatment options such as partial hospitalization and manualized psychotherapies—adds a further complication to this regulatory problem, as purchasers must develop strategies to match patients and provider types.

Finally, the confluence of all these factors—opportunities posed by developments outside mental health, a growing supply of diverse providers, and difficulties of regulatory control—promoted development of a wholly new institution in mental health care delivery, the managed behavioral health care carve-out, which has, by exploiting these features of the system, succeeded in reducing costs while expanding the number of people who obtain services. This new institution raises additional questions for public policy in mental health.

Changes in the Provision of Mental Health Services since 1950

In 1955, 322 state and county mental hospitals provided almost all inpatient services in the United States (US PCMH, 1978b; Grob 2001). These large, mainly isolated hospitals were staffed by a generally unskilled custodial staff and a relatively small staff of professional psychiatrists. Most private psychiatrists, some 85 percent, were in private practice, concentrated in a few urban markets (Mechanic, 1969). In 1954, for example, about 20 percent of all practicing psychiatrists in the United States were located on the island of Manhattan (Clausen, 1956). The supply of other mental health professionals was modest. In 1955 there were 13,500 psychologists and 20,000 members of the National Association of Social Workers; most of them did not provide mental health care.

State and county mental hospitals operated under the direct control of the state and county governments and were supervised by specialized bureaucracies. Under these arrangements, staff were often able to advance their own interests through their influence on the state government bureaucracy. This administrative system often protected patients only to the extent that their interests coincided with those of staff.

By 2000 the size and significance of this publicly operated supply system had declined substantially. Inpatient capacity, measured as total beds per capita, was only one-quarter as high in 1998 as it had been in 1955 (Manderscheid et al., 2001). The skill distribution of the mental health workforce has also changed. There are now proportionally fewer psychiatrists and many fewer unskilled workers, but substantially more college and master's level professionals (psychologists, social workers, and counselors). The number of psychologists and social workers has more than quadrupled (West et al., 2001). Whereas fifty years ago describing and estimating the supply of mental health services was largely a simple task consisting of counting public mental hospital beds and psychiatrists in solo office-based practice, today there is a complex and diverse set of institutions and professions in the business of treating mental disorders.

Inpatient Services

Figure 5.1 illustrates the evolution of the inpatient sector of specialty mental health supply over the period 1970–2000. It is important to note that this figure describes only changes in supply *within* the mental health sector. It does not capture those who left through the "back door" of the public mental hospital and were then reinstitutionalized in nursing homes and medical-surgical beds in general hospitals (sometimes referred to as scatter beds).

The thirty-year period before 1980 was characterized by an enormous decline in inpatient beds, entirely a consequence of shrinkage in the number of state, county, and Veterans Administration (VA) system beds. Most of the decline took the form of closing beds within institutions, rather than closing the institutions themselves. Large public mental health specialty institutions became less important as a source of service supply over this period primarily because they shrank

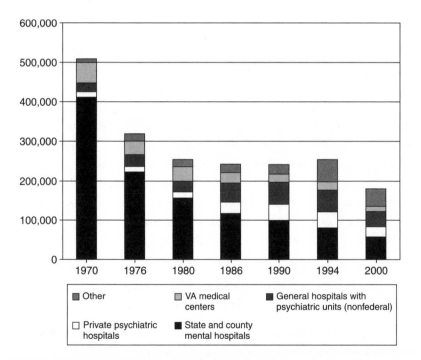

Figure 5.1. Distribution of Inpatient Beds for Mentally Ill Persons, by Type of Institution

SOURCE: Data from US DHHS, CMHS, 2004, chap. 18, table 2 (www.mentalhealth.samhsa.gov/publications/allpubs/SMA04-3938/chp18table2.asp).

disproportionately while other sectors grew slowly. Between 1970 and 1980 state and county hospitals lost more than 250,000 beds, while the sum of the increases in private psychiatric hospital beds and beds in other (non-VA) specialty institutions was quite small. Nonetheless, as late as 1980, and despite massive shrinkage, public hospitals dedicated to the care of people with mental illness continued to dominate the supply of institutional services.

Between 1980 and 2000 the total number of beds remained quite stable and only recently resumed a decline (to about 190,000 beds). In fact, for a period between 1986 and 1994 there was some growth in the number of psychiatric beds in the United States (Manderscheid et al., 2001). Yet underlying this stable trend was a marked shift in composition. The number of state, county, and VA hospital beds fell by a striking 60 percent, as institutions themselves closed. By contrast, private (primarily for-profit) hospital and general hospital psychiatric unit bed capacity grew by 85 to 90 percent through 1994. By the end of this period, from 1994 to 2000, private psychiatric hospital beds declined by 40 percent and general hospital beds by 28 percent. The overall result was a further decline in psychiatric beds.

In contrast to the slow decline in the number of public hospitals during the period of deinstitutionalization, a change in financial incentives for child hospitalization in the early 1990s and the rise of managed care led the number of for-profit hospitals to plummet. Between 1976 and 1992 the number of private psychiatric hospitals increased by nearly 300. In the six years between 1992 and 1998, the number fell by 125 (more than the total number of state and county mental hospitals that have closed since 1970). The rapid entry and exit of private institutions in the mental hospital market parallels a similar pattern in the medical market (Kessler and McClellan, 2002). Private for-profit hospitals, largely unconstrained by community and political pressure and able to obtain financing rapidly through capital markets, are much more responsive to changing incentives than are either public or not-for-profit providers.

General Health Policy Changes and the Supply of Institutional Services

In chapter 4 we described how changes in public programs—specifically the introduction of Medicaid—contributed to deinstitutionalization and to the shrinkage of the public hospital system. The subsequent growth of nonpublic institutional providers in the 1980s also stems from changes outside the mental health system.

In the 1980s national health policy moved to deregulate the hospital sector. Mounting evidence of the inefficiency of regulation, combined with an ideological shift favoring markets, led to changes at the state and federal levels. State certificate-of-need (CON) laws, which had served to regulate hospital capacity and capital intensity, began to be weakened or eliminated (Salkever, 2000). This deregulation of hospital capacity created opportunities for general and private psychiatric hospitals to meet the growing demand for mental health care that was in part fueled by the expansion of public and private insurance coverage for care of these illnesses (see chapter 4 and McGuire [1981] for more complete discussions of the expansion of insurance).

In the 1980s the federal government also replaced its existing hospital payment system for Medicare with the diagnosis-related group (DRG) prospective payment system. Under DRGs, length of stay declined and hospital occupancy rates began to drop sharply. Many general hospitals opened psychiatric units in the 1980s so that psychiatric patients could fill otherwise empty beds and to avoid the DRG system because psychiatric units were offered an exemption from the system.

Public financing changes also contributed to the pattern of institutional change. Rules permitting states to use Medicaid dollars to pay for the care of juvenile and elderly beneficiaries in psychiatric hospitals created an entirely new revenue stream for these institutions. Thus, the ability to increase capacity, coupled with insurance mechanisms that expanded demand, led to growth in the supply of psychiatric inpatient providers.

Analyses of private insurance and Medicaid spending showed especially large increases in inpatient psychiatric treatment of children during the 1980s that accounted for a disproportionate fraction of the rate of growth in mental health spending (Frank et al., 1991). The increase in the supply and use of private, for-profit psychiatric hospital inpatient services was particularly striking for children—among children hospitalized for psychiatric disorders in short-stay institutions, nearly one-quarter were hospitalized in for-profit proprietary institutions. Likewise, length of stay for children in general hospital psychiatric units clearly responded to the generous financial incentives of this period.

Institutional Convergence

The public mental hospital of the beginning of this period had an identifiable and unique character (whether for good or ill). It provided treatment and some custodial services to a population of acutely ill patients, many of whom would be discharged after short stays, and custodial services, with minimal treatment, to a population of chronically ill patients, most of whom would spend very long periods in the institution. Its staff consisted of a small number—often a very small number—of professional mental health workers and a large number of less skilled custodial workers. An extreme example of this, Bryce Hospital in Alabama (the institution that provoked the lawsuit in *Wyatt v. Stickney*), housed 5,200 patients and had a staff of 1,500. That staff's professional component included just one doctoral-trained psychologist, three physicians (none of them psychiatrists), and two MSWs. Though Bryce was an outlier, even nationally as late as 1970 there was only about one psychiatrist per one hundred inpatient beds in state and county mental hospitals (Manderscheid et al., 2001). A typical hospital was very large and often incorporated all the services of a small town. The unusual nature of this institution is exemplified by the extensive literature about the interactions between its patients and staff. Few other modern institutions would yield a comparable literature.

State and county hospitals were quite different from the other institutional service providers of this period. Private psychiatric hospitals were much smaller and much more focused on treatment. A large share of their caseload consisted of patients with neurotic disorders who were less severely ill. General hospital psychiatric units were smaller still; they primarily served acutely ill patients and did not share the custodial functions of state and county hospitals. Over the past three decades these three previously distinct types of institutions have converged in size, staffing patterns, length of stay, and patient mix. Today it is more difficult to delineate their unique functions. The growing similarities among these institutions give public and private payers, and patients, more options in terms of both cost and quality.

State, county, and VA hospitals have shrunk dramatically—the average number of beds per institution fell by 80 percent, to an average of about 270, in 2000. The private psychiatric hospital sector, in which the number of institutions fluctuated wildly in the 1980s and 1990s, consistently maintained an average size of about 100 beds per institution. The number of general hospitals offering inpatient psychiatric units has expanded, but their size has remained quite stable over time at about 35 beds (ibid.).

Convergence also occurred in staffing. Professional staff per bed has always been much higher in general hospital psychiatric units and private psychiatric hospitals than in state hospitals, which continue to provide more custodial services. Substantial differences in the use of professionals across different types of psychiatric institutions persist. But the differences have been shrinking over

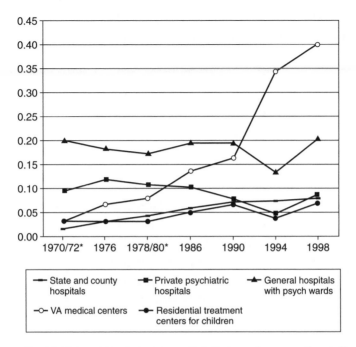

Figure 5.2. Psychiatrists and Psychologists per Bed. Beds are from 1970/80; staff are from 1972/78.

SOURCE: Data from US DHHS, CMHS, 2004, chap. 18, tables 2 and 7a–7f (www.mentalhealth.samhsa. gov/publications/allpubs/SMA04-3938/chp18.asp).

time (fig. 5.2) as professional staff per bed rose in public facilities and fell in private hospitals and general hospitals.

Reductions in average size and increases in professional staffing were a necessary corollary of the pattern of deinstitutionalization of the 1970s and 1980s. States reduced the number of beds within institutions but shied away from politically more volatile acts of closing institutions and laying off staff. Court-ordered staffing levels, such as those specified in *Wyatt v. Stickney,* also forced states to maintain staffing even while reducing occupancy. Indeed, reductions in beds were often accomplished without any losses in staff positions. For example, while the number of beds in state and county mental hospitals decreased by 31 percent from 1986 to 1994, total staff decreased by 18.5 percent. Even in the 1990s, when states finally did close public mental hospitals, average bed count continued to fall and average staffing ratios continued to rise. In 1994 there were nearly 25 percent more psychiatrists and psychologists per bed in state and county mental hospitals than in 1986.

Lengths of stay were also converging. In 1970 the median length of stay for admissions to state hospitals was 41 days. By 1975, although this figure had fallen to 25 days, it still far exceeded length of stay in general hospitals. In 1988 the median length of stay for a terminated patient was 9.9 days in private, nonprofit hospitals and 12.6 in state and county hospitals. But by 1994 median length of stay in state and county hospitals was virtually identical to that in private, nonprofit institutions. Public mental hospitals have lost their custodial character and, like other institutional providers, primarily offer a setting for the provision of acute-care services.

Although the composition of the inpatient caseload continues to differ among institution types, even the most seriously ill patients are now seen in a variety of institutional settings. In 1970, for example, about 42 percent of hospital admission of patients with schizophrenia occurred in state and county hospitals (fig. 5.3). By 1997 fewer than 20 percent of these hospitalizations took place in public hospitals. Both general hospital units and private psychiatric hospitals had increased their share of this market. Functional differences among institutions do remain. State and county mental hospitals' patients continue to be more seriously and chronically ill than those at other types of institutions. These institutions also continue to protect the public from forensic patients.

Provider Diversity through New Institutional Arrangements: Intermediate Facilities

Complementing the diversity of providers offering inpatient psychiatric care, entirely new institutions have arisen to provide alternatives to this care. Such alternative institutional arrangements include CMHCs (discussed in chapter 4) and partial hospitalization. By 1970 more than seven hundred institutions nationally offered partial-care services, and within six years the number of these institutions had nearly doubled, in part because of requirements that CMHCs include these services. An early review of the cost-effectiveness of partial hospitalization noted that there had never been "an unsuccessful effort to discover alternative treatment—[alternatives are] always as good as hospitalization and always less expensive" (Segal and Kotler, 1989).

A recent review confirms this result (Horvitz-Lennon et al., 2001). Partial hospitalization appears to be as effective as full hospitalization in providing basic care to adults with moderate mental disorders (ibid.). Patient and family satisfaction and social functioning are typically better under partial hospitalization. Rehospitalization rates are similar for both care settings. But for the same type

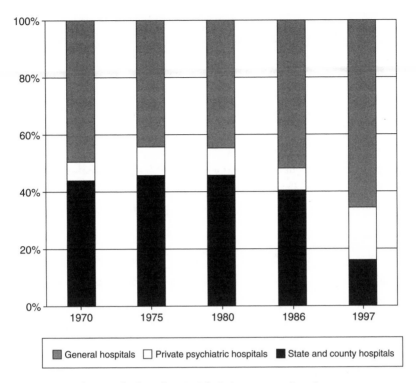

Figure 5.3. Distribution of Schizophrenia Admissions among Inpatients
SOURCE: Data from US DHHS, CMHS, *Mental Health, U.S.,* 1983–2000.

of patient, partial hospitalization is less expensive than full hospitalization (ibid). Sledge and his colleagues (1996) estimated an average of 20 percent cost saving per patient by using partial care.

The number of institutions offering partial hospitalization services has grown steadily, albeit a little more slowly recently, since 1976. At first, the growth of partial hospitalization was stymied by the difficulty of developing new sources of funds to cover alternative treatment modalities. Now that the cost-effectiveness of this modality has been amply demonstrated (at least for certain populations), Medicaid and Medicare both pay for partial hospitalization in instances where they would otherwise pay for inpatient services. Even so, the reallocation of state funds from the state hospitals to partial hospitalization programs is slow and complicated by the variations among states in mental health care funding (Dickey et al., 1989).

One reason for this slow progress has to do with the pattern of diffusion of partial hospitalization (a problem common to other hospital alternatives and to many medical treatments as well). A treatment alternative is often assessed by its effectiveness for a specific population. In practice, however, a program often diffuses more broadly; it may be used both for the originally intended population and for populations that are sicker and healthier than the original group. Partial care services appear to be cost-effective when used for moderately severely ill patients. They may not be cost-effective with respect to the efficiency of the whole system if they diffuse to other populations. Yet the growth of Medicaid and Medicare funding appears to have generated precisely this outcome, as partial care programs are used as fiscally but not clinically efficient alternatives to long-term hospitalization (Hogan, 1981). The diffusion of technologies in both directions, combined with the heterogeneity of populations, makes it difficult to set prices for alternatives appropriately.

Professional Services

Public and private interest in expanding the supply of mental health professionals began in the immediate post–World War II period, as planners and professional leaders recognized the potential for providing services in the community. Faced with a shortage of psychiatrists and the return of thousands of veterans with psychiatric disorders, the newly created National Institute of Mental Health (NIMH) invested in training to ensure an adequate supply of professionals capable of treating problems. The VA also supported training programs at university departments of psychology.

Before World War II psychologists rarely delivered direct patient care; rather, they worked as researchers and conducted assessments. The growth of the profession of clinical psychology began immediately after the war. In 1945 and 1946 Connecticut certified and Virginia then licensed individuals to practice psychology. Shortly after, NIMH sponsored a training conference and began to offer training grants (Reinehr, 1975). In 1958, 572 Americans received doctorates in psychology. By 1978, 3,055 psychology doctorates were awarded. By 1998 there were nearly 77,000 licensed clinical psychologists (fig. 5.4).

The social work profession has a longer history, dating back to the mid-nineteenth century. In 1958, however, fewer than 1,750 people were awarded an MSW, and most of them did not have counseling training. In 1978, 9,500 MSWs were awarded, and twenty years later, nearly 14,000. Today the vast majority of social workers provide direct patient care rather than being involved in research, teaching, or administration.

The fourth mental health professionals, psychiatric nurses, had always worked in psychiatric hospitals, but the development of specialized training in psychiat-

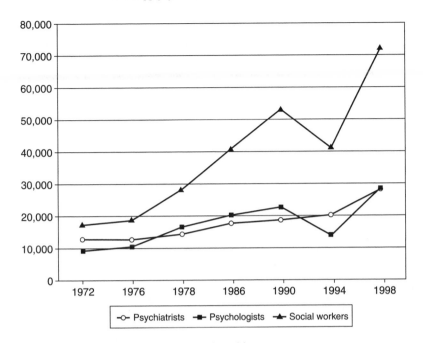

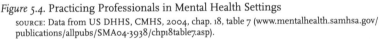

Figure 5.4. Practicing Professionals in Mental Health Settings
SOURCE: Data from US DHHS, CMHS, 2004, chap. 18, table 7 (www.mentalhealth.samhsa.gov/ publications/allpubs/SMA04-3938/chp18table7.asp).

ric nursing is a relatively new phenomenon. In 1968, 327 people graduated with degrees in psychiatric nursing. By 1978 the number had doubled. In 1995, 6,800 nurses were certified as specialists in psychiatric-mental health nursing (West et al., 2001).

Finally, the counseling profession grew dramatically as a result of the Community Mental Health Centers Act of 1963. Today it is the largest mental health professional group, with more than 108,000 counselors licensed by states or by the National Board for Certified Counselors.

Although governmental funding and interest date back to the 1940s, between 1950 and about 1964 there was little change in the number of those in the main mental health professions. Between 1964 and 1976, by contrast, there was explosive growth in the supply of nonpsychiatrist mental health professionals. Entry into these professions then flattened out between 1976 and 1990. After 1990 graduation from master's level programs took off once again, but growth in PhD psychology graduates stagnated.

Figure 5.5 illustrates the evolution of these fields since 1950 using data on new trainees. To improve comparability, the figure describes training using data

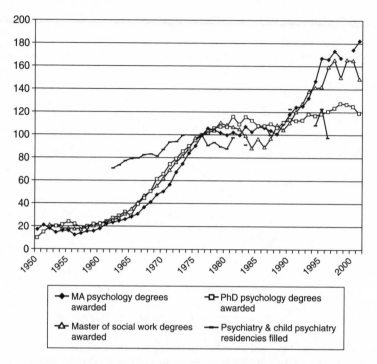

Figure 5.5. Indexed Number of Trainees for Mental Health Professions (1976 = 100)
SOURCES: Data from Lindsay, 1982; NSF, 2004, table 50 (www.nsf.gov/statistics/nsf04311/tables/tab50.xls);
Council on Social Work Education (1977, 1998); NIMH, *Mental Health, U.S.,* 1983, table 5.3; US DHHS,
CMHS, *Mental Health, U.S.,* 1992, table 5.2; US DHHS, CMHS, *Mental Health, U.S.,* 1996, table 10.8.

indexed to 100 in 1976. In 1976 there were 7,859 master's degrees awarded in psychology, 2,883 doctorates awarded in psychology, 9,080 master's degrees awarded in social work, and 4,938 residents in psychiatry and child psychiatry (Council on Social Work Education, 1977; NSF, 2004; AMA, *Directory of Graduate Medical Education Programs,* various years).

Strikingly, entry into psychiatry residency programs lagged both the other mental health professions and medical care more generally (not shown), increasing only 75 percent over this period. In 1963 there were only about 60 percent as many active psychologists as psychiatrists; by 1997 there were more than twice as many active psychologists as psychiatrists. There has been little change in hours worked on average by psychiatrists over this period.

Finally, within the medical sector, generalist physicians now provide a somewhat greater share of mental health services. In 1977 about 28 percent of all physician visits with a mental health diagnosis were to generalists; by 1997 this figure had increased to 34 percent. (These figures are our tabulations of National Center for Health Statistics, National Ambulatory Medical Care Survey.)

Supply and Incentives

What drove these changes in training? The postwar period saw substantial increases in college and graduate training throughout the economy. Similarly, the size of the baby boom cohort meant that when its members began higher education, the number of newly trained professionals increased rapidly. But neither of these cohortwide effects can explain most of the growth in the number of mental health professionals. The increase in skilled mental health workers came after the GI bill had its effect and before the baby boomers reached graduate school. NIMH funding for professional training in mental health helped, but roughly half of this funding went toward psychiatric training, and there was little increase in the supply of psychiatrists. The VA, as noted earlier, aggressively invested in psychology training programs. The development of CMHCs, which hired mental health professionals in the community, generated a new source of demand. CMHCs employed many of these new trainees (between 1972 and 1976 CMHCs hired 29.5 percent of newly trained psychiatrists and 47.1 percent of newly trained psychologists), but deinstitutionalization offset some of this increment. Most of the new professionals were not employed in designated mental health institutions. Many of them were in private practice, and many were employed outside traditional mental health settings.

Instead, we find that these changes in supply were prompted by the high rates of economic return to investments in training in these mental health professions in an era of expanding financing. We examined rates of return from professional training in mental health fields using data from the census and from the AMA. The data suggest that supply does respond to rates of return. For example, when rates of return from training in psychiatry (compared to training in general practice) have been high (10%), the number of psychiatry residencies filled in the subsequent years tended to increase. The data for psychology and social work reflect degrees awarded, not programs entered, so the correspondence is less precise.

Looking at the pattern of rates of return, we find that the data suggest that the economic returns from training in psychology in the early postwar period were about 10 to 25 percent above the returns from a BA, which prompted increased entry into the psychology profession. Economic rates of return have been falling since about 1970, which is consistent with the flattening out of supply. In fact, by 2000 the returns were generally negative; that is, economic returns from a mental health profession were lower than those from an alternative occupational choice. The large numbers of newly trained psychologists and social workers entering the profession by 1970 probably depressed returns for those who followed them.

Influencing the Political Process

In the era when public mental hospitals dominated the provision of mental health services, the staff of these institutions had a powerful political voice. In the public system, deinstitutionalization occurred through closures of beds in specific hospitals. Enormous numbers of beds closed, however, before institutions themselves began to close entirely. The political economy of institutional closure depended not only on patients, but also on local community and staff interests. Just as patients received custodial care in the total institution, staff received civil service employment from those institutions, which often were located in rural areas, where there were few other sources of employment (Goldman, 1977). State mental health authority bureaucrats established strong ties to these institutions, and decisions to close beds or institutions often faced fierce and effective political resistance.

Psychiatrists, like the rest of the medical profession, benefited by limiting professional entry through public licensure. For many years, psychiatrists even closed the psychoanalytic training system to nonmedical professionals. As they grew, the newer mental health professions — psychology, social work, psychiatric nursing, and counseling — also employed the political process to strengthen their economic position. Such behavior was particularly important in the period after 1970, when the rates of return to education in these professions began to decline. State licensing laws established education and training standards and codes of professional conduct. These were necessary conditions for fully recognized professions that would be delegated the task of self-regulation by the states.

Licensure was the first step to gaining access to insurance reimbursement. In the 1960s psychologists and social workers could be reimbursed by insurance only indirectly—through a physician. Organized psychology invested heavily in political campaigns to enact so-called freedom of choice laws that required direct reimbursement of the psychologist as an independent professional. Social workers pursued what became known as vendorship statutes that permitted social workers to be directly reimbursed. The first such law passed in New Jersey in 1967; by 1990 forty-two states had passed such laws. Likewise, in its 1972 decision the Montgomery federal court in *Wyatt v. Stickney* defined the term "skilled mental health professional" to include a psychiatrist, a doctoral-trained psychologist, a master's degree social worker with two years of experience, or an RN with a graduate degree and two years of experience.

Over the next decades, influenced by the political clout of the diverse mental health professional associations, legislatures around the country passed mandates that required insurers to cover mental health services provided by these professionals. These laws were buttressed by antitrust suits filed against insurers who refused to cover mental health services provided by psychologists (*Blue Shield of Virginia v. McCready*, 475 U.S. 465 [1982]). Table 5.1 shows the states that passed mandates through the 1970s and 1980s. The final barrier concerned training in psychoanalysis. Psychoanalytic institutes had historically restricted their training to psychiatrists and zealously guarded their turf. By the early 1990s, however, they too were forced to open their doors to doctorally trained psychologists and came under pressure to accept social workers as well.

The latest effort to maintain the earnings of psychologists has been the fight to grant them prescribing privileges. The fact that opposition to such efforts has come primarily from psychiatrists suggests that, despite the divergence in the training of these professionals, they view each other as direct competition.

Competition among Professionals

In the 1970s and 1980s both the supply of and demand for professional mental health services expanded. Financing and regulatory changes promoted the growth and diversity of supply. Moreover, payment policies in this period relied on the use of prevailing usual, customary, and reasonable (UCR) fee schedules to pay all professionals. The consequence was that though there was some competition for patients among providers, they generally did not compete on price.

Figure 5.6 shows earnings per hour for psychologists, social workers, and psychiatrists. The figure suggests that earnings move in parallel for the professions outside psychiatry, from which it can be inferred that the same forces influence them all.

Despite the lack of explicit price competition, the growing supply of licensed providers across diverse fields has reduced the hourly earnings of the most costly provider groups. Laws enabling nonpsychiatrists to compete directly with psychiatrists placed downward pressure on the earnings of psychiatrists (see fig. 5.6 and Frank [1985] for an economic explanation). Similarly, over time the gap between psychologists' earnings and those of psychiatric social workers has grown smaller.

The existence of a diverse array of providers gives policy makers opportunities to generate competition among them and, as the Supreme Court suggested in its decision in *Olmstead* (see chapter 6), to provide better, less restrictive care opportunities. Ultimately, this competition generates lower prices and efficient organizational forms. Thus, for example, if counselors are able to provide mental health

TABLE 5.1.
Regulation of Mental Health Services Insurance, by State

State	Mandate Type — Mandated Benefits Package	Mandate Type — Mandated Availability	Year	Services Covered — Inpatient	Services Covered — Outpatient	Services Covered — Partial Hospitalization	Policies Covered — Group	Policies Covered — Individual
Arkansas	X		1979	X	X		X	X
California		X	1973	X	X		X	
Colorado	X		1976	X	X	X	X	
Connecticut	X		1971	X	X	X	X	X
Florida		X	1976/83	X	X	X	X	
Georgia		X	1984	X	X		X	X
Illinois		X	1975	X	X		X	X
Kansas		X	1978	X	X		X	X
Louisiana		X	1975	X	X		X	
Maine	X		1983	X	X		X	
Maryland	X		1974	X	X		X	X
Massachusetts	X		1973	X	X		X	X
Minnesota	X		1975	X	X		X	
Missouri		X	1980	X	X		X	X
Montana	X		1983	X	X		X	
New Hampshire	X		1975	X	X	X	X	
New York		X	1977	X	X		X	
North Dakota	X		1975	X		X	X	
Ohio	X		1978		X		X	
Oregon			1984	X	X	X	X	
Tennessee		X	1974		X		X	
Vermont		X	1975	X	X	X	X	
Virginia	X		1975	X			X	X
Washington		X	1983				X	
West Virginia		X	1977	X	X		X	X
Wisconsin	X		1975/85	X	X		X	

SOURCE: Frank, 1989, 127.

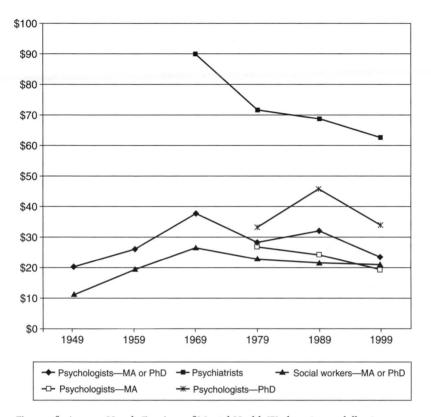

Figure 5.6. Average Hourly Earnings of Mental Health Workers (2002 dollars)
SOURCES: Data from U.S. Census (1950, 1960, 1970, 1980, 1990, 2000); AMA, *Profile of Medical Practice* (1982, 1983, 1987, 1993, 1999); AMA, *Physician Socioeconomic Statistics* (2000–2002); AMA, *Socioeconomic Characteristics of Medical Practice* (1979, 1980); AMA, *Physician Marketplace Statistics* (1995, 1997–98); AMA, *Physician Characteristics and Distribution in the US* (1981, 1983, 1986, 1987, 1990, 1993, 1994, 1996–97, 1997–98, 1999, 2000–2001).

services as effectively as more highly trained professionals, they should displace the latter from the market. The existence of a large and diverse array of suppliers also increases the benefit of using flexible forms of funding and of intermediaries who can exploit variations in payment and efficiency (Sturm and Klap, 1999).

Institutional Response: The Rise of Managed Behavioral Health Care

The rapid expansion of inpatient psychiatric treatment capacity in the 1980s, propelled by deregulation and expanded insurance coverage, led to growth in mental health spending that exceeded overall growth in health care spending

(Bruzzese, 1989; Ferguson, 1990; Williams, 1990). The popular press was filled with scandalous accounts of psychiatric hospital chains paying bounty hunters to generate adolescent admissions from local general hospital emergency rooms (where teenagers with substance abuse and emotional problems were often provided with acute treatment). At the same time, managed care, an organizational alternative to traditional health insurance, was gaining interest among health care payers. Mental health care, and inpatient care, seemed an ideal setting for managing health care (Feldman, 2003). A specialized set of managed care organizations rapidly responded to the demand for specialized expertise in containing mental health care spending, which led to the birth of the managed behavioral health care carve-out industry.[1]

Specialty carve-out managed behavioral health organizations (MBHOs) immediately aimed to reduce admission rates and durations of treatment for inpatient psychiatric care. They implemented care management processes such as prior authorization screening of psychiatric admissions. This rapidly reduced admission rates, which left excess capacity for inpatient psychiatric care. For example, in 1986—a year before the large-scale introduction of MBHOs—occupancy rates in private psychiatric hospitals averaged 72 percent. Eight years later, in 1994, when managed care dominated the industry, occupancy rates in private psychiatric hospitals had declined to 63 percent, where they remain today.[2] Unlike most public purchasers, MBHOs could easily redirect patients toward facilities that offered attractive prices. In combination with the availability of capacity, this ability to direct volume gave MBHOs the upper hand in negotiations with hospitals over price. The mid-1990s saw the first contraction in the size of private psychiatric hospitals since the 1960s and real declines in inpatient spending.

The growth of MBHOs also altered the environment for professional providers. MBHOs recognized that for many mental health problems a range of professions could be equally effective in treatment. By directing patients to less costly types of providers, they could expand the number of people receiving services while reducing costs. Furthermore, they could use their ability to direct patient volume to sign up professionals despite offering reduced fees. The results of this two-pronged approach are reflected in Figure 5.6: earnings for psychologists and psychiatrists declined during the 1990s, whereas those of social workers remained roughly constant.

Certainly, MBHOs have not been the first institution to attempt to tame costs in the mental health marketplace. Public and private purchasers have always been concerned about the cost of mental health services. Until the advent of MBHOs, however, the principal method for regulating costs was through administratively setting price and fee schedules. It is very difficult to establish and maintain administrative fee schedules so as to exploit competitive forces and overcapacities, particularly in a world of heterogeneous populations and technological change. Under administered pricing, policy makers must assign differentials to diverse providers on the basis of an assessment of their efficiency. Increases in supply may not generate compensating declines in price. Pricing (whether market or administered) is also more difficult when services must be delivered to heterogeneous populations. This is especially true in the case of bundled payment arrangements, such as case-based or capitation payments, where failure to compensate providers for treating sicker patients will result in healthy patients crowding out sicker ones. By combining pricing strategies with explicit management efforts, including directing patients to preferred facilities and providers, MBHOs have been far more successful than earlier institutions in controlling costs within the mental health service system.

To date the evidence suggests that for the most part these reductions in spending and costs have not come at the expense of the quality of care. This is consistent with the existence of system overcapacity in the period before the entry of MBHOs. As this overcapacity is exhausted, however, the challenge will be to retain the cost-control advantages of MBHOs without excessively curtailing the quality of care.

Conclusions

Public policy (through regulation and financing), coupled with expanded private insurance, has had powerful effects on the supply of mental health care. These policy changes expanded insurance coverage and gave most Americans the financial ability to obtain mental health care provided by a range of professionals and institutions. This growth in the funding available for mental health services also encouraged institutions and individuals to provide the services that this funding would then reimburse. They led to the development of a large, diverse, robust, and competitive market for mental health professional and institutional services.

This expansion of supply, in turn, generated growth in mental health spending, growth that was often viewed as extreme. By the late 1980s mental health care outdistanced most other areas of medical care in spending growth. Existing regulatory mechanisms—particularly administered fee schedules—were inadequate to address these cost pressures.

The market responded. The 1990s brought on the era of managed care, at the insistence of large payers (including Medicaid). Specialized MBHOs took advantage of the substantial available capacity and potential competition among provider groups to create an era of price competition that significantly affected the economic prospects of mental health professionals and institutions alike. Mental health spending has slowed, professional incomes have fallen, and for the first time in a generation the number of private psychiatric beds has declined. By 2000 consumers were actually paying less for many key mental health services than they had been in the late 1980s.

The expansion in supply and diversity of mental health services throughout this period has, in itself, been a benefit to consumers. It has been particularly useful combined with the move toward insurance-based financing, through which consumers have more choice over their care. The consumer in 2000 had, by historical standards, a vast array of well-trained professionals and institutions from which to obtain treatment. Access to mental health care is greater for most people than has been true before. The advent of MBHOs, which direct patients to panels and limit use, has restricted choice somewhat but has produced substantial cost savings to offset these restrictions. By inducing competition and bringing costs down, MBHOs have helped consumers gain the full advantage of this expanded supply system.

CHAPTER 6

Policy Making in Mental Health

Integration, Mainstreaming, and Shifting Institutions

In the 1950s and 1960s mental health policy making was the domain of governors and their state mental health program directors. Organized psychiatry wielded great influence and was deeply involved in consequential debates about the future of mental health care in the United States. Today, by contrast, state Medicaid directors, the Social Security commissioner, the administrator of the Centers for Medicare and Medicaid Services (CMS), and human resource directors in U.S. corporations are the voices with the greatest influence on the direction of mental health policy. These policy makers have little direct connection with the specialty mental health sector. Many of their offices did not even exist in 1950. They are mainstream policy makers. The decline of mental health exceptionalism in public policy has been accompanied by a parallel decline in exceptionalism in policy making.

Mental Health Policy Making at Midcentury

In the 1950s mental health policy was primarily the responsibility of the states, who also paid for most care (Fein, 1958). Most of this funding was allocated to the activities of the public mental hospital, and these hospitals were managed by psychiatrists. The people most directly associated with the direction and management of mental health care were in state government, closely linked to the profession of psychiatry.

In the aftermath of World War II, a sizable number of psychiatrists developed the belief that the mental hospital should no longer be the central institution of the mental health care system. This increasingly popular view of mental health delivery began to weaken the links among state government, the state hospital, and the profession of psychiatry. Organized psychiatry debated the direction of mental health delivery throughout the 1950s. Community-based psychiatry gained the upper hand through the leadership of psychiatrists such as Robert Rappaport, Harry Solomon, and Walter Barton.

The initial reforms that began to reorient mental health care in the United States emanated from the states and from state organizations such as the Governors Conference and the Council of State Governments (Grob, 2001). Individual states such as New York, California, and Massachusetts were among the first to adopt policies that began to shift resources in the direction of community-based mental health services. These states created grant programs with incentives for the development and expansion of community-based mental health clinics, albeit with modest funding. Other states followed suit, and during the 1950s there was a dramatic expansion in the number of outpatient mental health clinics, the majority of which were funded by state government. This growth in community clinics was driven in part by a belief in community-based treatment and by the hope that such care would reduce reliance on expensive state mental hospitals.

State officials and their ideas were also central to efforts aimed at identifying mental health care as a nationwide problem that had to be addressed in consistent policy terms. For example, when the Joint Commission on Mental Illness and Health (JCMIH) was created in the 1950s by a set of private interest groups and philanthropic organizations, the director of the commission was Jack Ewalt, the mental health commissioner in Massachusetts. The 1950s and early 1960s were a time when mental health became a matter for national policy. The creation of the National Institute of Mental Health in the late 1940s gave mental health policy a voice in the federal government. Technical specialists, such as the NIMH director Robert Felix, influenced the emerging federal interest in mental illness from the perspective of the specialty mental health sector. The policy statements that resulted from this initial effort of developing a national approach to mental health policy were based on ideas emerging from the professions and the states.[1] The JCMIH pointed to a two-pronged strategy for improving mental health care. One prong involved improving the conditions and the treatment capacity of public mental hospitals; the other worked at developing a community-based system of care primarily aimed at people with severe mental disorders.

Federal mental health policy until 1963 was limited to establishing a bully pulpit that helped activate a variety of interests to work on altering the directions of mental health care in the United States. The federal government's expanding role in social insurance and in civil rights contributed to a view that it might work in concert with localities to fix mental health care and avoid the political clout associated with interests linked to state mental hospitals. At this point, state interests and proponents of community mental health care began to part company on matters of federal policy. The shape of the new community mental health centers (CMHC) legislation emphasized new institutions that bypassed states by forming federal-local partnerships based on financing arrangements that mimicked the Hill-Burton hospital expansion program (the 1946 federal initiative that funded the expansion of hospital beds in the United States).[2] The NIMH was given responsibility for managing the new CMHC program. Yet, while a shift was taking place regarding what shape the mental health system would take, the debate stayed primarily within the mental health community.

This growing federal interest was not accompanied by a massive injection of funds. States remained the main funders of mental health services. State officials such as Ewalt, Milton Greenblatt, and others continued to have great influence on the shape of mental health delivery.

Watershed Events in Mental Health Policy: Medicaid, Medicare, and SSI

The launch of President Johnson's Great Society initiative in 1964 unleashed forces that would fundamentally change mental health care financing and delivery in the United States—and the political institutions that had shaped mental health policy. The passage of Medicaid, Medicare, and later the Supplemental Security Income (SSI) program greatly expanded the resources available to treat mental illness. These programs made the federal government a much more significant payer and regulator of mental health care. At the same time, they began to take mental health policy making out of the hands of the mental health sector.

The debate over coverage of mental health care under Medicare offered the first indication that powerful new institutions were being created that would exert great influence over the care of people with mental illness, yet the mental health community would have only a modest say over what would emerge. Before the implementation of Medicare, organized psychiatry engaged in a series of attempts to influence the new program's design. During the debate in 1965, the modern argument over parity in insurance benefits for mental health care first surfaced. The mental health community called on Congress to abandon the practices of the private health insurance sector and offer comprehensive and comparable insurance benefits for mental health care and other medical care under the Medicare program. The arguments for equal treatment of mental health care were based on fairness—that it is wrong to discriminate against people with mental disorders. The arguments against equal coverage took aim at the difficulties in defining mental illness, the lack of evidence of effective treatments, the high costs of covering mental health services, and the uncertainty in making actuarial cost estimates (Frank, 2000). Congress chose to follow the private health insurance market as a model for choosing nearly all features of the benefit design under Medicare, including mental health. Concerns with the program's budget, disruption of existing health care arrangements, and program administration won the day.

The American Psychiatric Association's preparation for the implementation of the Medicare program also illustrated the new political and organizational context within which psychiatry (and mental health groups generally) had to operate in order to affect mental health policy. The specialty mental health concerns in policy were increasingly focused on preserving benefits in the context of a larger policy-making apparatus whose agenda reached far beyond issues of mental health care. The enactment of Medicare was accompanied by a new set of regulatory standards. Accreditation by the Joint Commission on Accreditation of Hospitals (JCAH, known today as JCAHO) was a central feature of quality assurance in Medicare. At the time, even though the JCAH had adopted APA standards for accreditation of psychiatric facilities, 33 percent of general hospitals and 66 percent of psychiatric hospitals were not accredited. The APA also proposed that a psychiatrist be appointed to the health insurance and medical review advisory councils for the Medicare program.

The ambulatory mental health benefit in Medicare carried high levels of cost sharing and strict limits on service utilization, so its immediate impact was muted. Mental health in Medicare remained a small share of Medicare spending for decades after its enactment. The late 1980s saw some expansion in Medicare coverage of care for mental disorders. Limits on psychotherapy were relaxed, the range of providers that could independently treat mental disorders was expanded to include psychologists and social workers, and a partial-hospital benefit was added. These changes resulted in expanded use of services and spending for mental health care (Rosenbach and Ammering, 1997).

Medicaid was similar to Medicare in terms of the role of the mental health community in policy making, but it had very different effects on mental health delivery. The program's focus on the poor and disabled and on the provision of long-term care for elderly persons meant that it included substantial numbers of people with mental illnesses who had previously relied on state mental health agencies for their care. The poor elderly mentally ill population was dramatically affected by the enactment of Medicaid. In 1963 there were 148,842 residents of state mental hospitals aged sixty-five or older, who accounted for 41 percent of all residents. By 1969, four years after the enactment of Medicaid, the number of these residents had declined to 111,420, or 22.7 percent of all residents (Kramer, 1977). During this same period the population of nursing homes nearly doubled. Following the enactment of Medicaid states faced a choice between hospitalizing indigent elderly people with dementia—and paying 100 percent of the costs in state mental hospitals—and placing them in nursing homes—and paying 17 percent to 50 percent of the costs (nursing homes also had lower per diem rates).

For poor and disabled people (after 1972) under age sixty-five, Medicaid also provided a form of health insurance for treatment of mental disorders, which was paid for under Medicaid's basic benefit. Again the costs to states of providing mental health services in the context of Medicaid were low. This presented strong inducements to mental health directors attempting to meet the mental health needs of their states under tight budgets to expand services by shifting priorities toward Medicaid-eligible populations and services covered by Medicaid. Of course, this strategy required that state mental health spending be applied to the state Medicaid match. As Medicaid grew to become the nation's largest mental health care payer, an increasingly large share of state mental health funds were being directly linked to Medicaid dollars.

Although Medicaid quickly became a central source of mental health funding, mental health concerns did not strongly influence Medicaid policy making. This lack of influence was noted in recommendations made by President Carter's Commission on Mental Health. The first recommendation of the Panel on Cost and Financing noted, "Stronger Federal leadership is needed with regard to the Medicaid mental health programs. This includes: Providing States with technical assistance in developing comprehensive mental health plans" (US PCMH, 1978b). The largest payer for mental health care in the United States was simply not attuned to mental health issues, in part because state mental health agencies were generally not a central part of the Medicaid policy-making process.

During the 1980s and 1990s state mental health agencies showed great creativity in developing ways of capturing more federal funds to pay for mental health care. Each new success added more funds to the public mental health care budget while state mental health policy makers surrendered ever more discretion over whom would be served and with what services (Frank et al., 2003). The result was that state mental health agencies could exercise less and less stewardship over mental health care for the poor and disadvantaged in their states.

Beginning in the 1960s, the period of introduction of Medicare and Medicaid, the federal government also introduced and expanded federal social insurance programs—Supplemental Security Income (SSI) and Social Security Disability Insurance (SSDI) offer income supports for disabled populations.

The introduction of these programs complemented Medicaid's effects in facilitating the shift of people with mental illness to the community. But state welfare agencies administer SSI, following federal rules. The federal Social Security Administration has authority over SSDI, and the federal Center for Medicare and Medicaid Services (formerly the Health Care Financing Administration) administers Medicare. Thus, the shift toward these programs also led to the creation of a new set of bureaucracies that were lifelines for people with mental illness but had little understanding of the unique aspects of creating community-based care and support of people with severe mental illnesses. Overall, mental health policy associated with Medicare, Medicaid, SSI, and SSDI was largely the by-product of policy aimed at health and disability insurance generally.

The federal block grant to state mental health agencies is the only remaining federal source of discretionary funds to these agencies. The Substance Abuse and Mental Health Services Administration (SAMHSA) controls the block grant. SAMHSA's staff is made up of experts in mental health care and substance abuse treatment delivery. The advisory councils are populated by people representing specialty providers, state mental health agencies, the mental health professions (e.g., psychiatry, social work, and psychology), managed behavioral health care industry representatives, and academics with specialized expertise in mental health. It has expertise—but few resources.

The Development of Mental Health Law

The judicial system represents yet another broad social institution that makes significant mental health policy decisions. Mental health law was a fledgling specialty area fifty years ago; it largely comprised cases concerning the insanity defense in criminal proceedings. Treatment was rarely a question brought before courts. Since then, the courts (both federal and state) have intervened, assuring people with mental illness new rights in the areas of involuntary commitment, civil competency, and treatment choice. The result has been that the conduct of mental hospitals, the autonomy of consumers, and the nature of provider-patient interactions have been shaped by courts. Commitment cases concern the balancing of individual and state interests as well as the risks of failing to commit and the risks of erroneous deprivation of liberty. The courts have established rights for people with serious mental disorders. One early case involving involuntary commitment (*Baxstrom v. Herald*, 383 U.S. 107 [1966]) extended equal protection rights under the Fourteenth Amendment to persons with mental illness. In a 1972 case (*Lessard v. Schmidt*, 349 F. Supp. 1078 [ED Wisconsin 1972]) the court found that civil commitment is at least as serious a deprivation of liberty as criminal confinement, and that a psychiatrist, when questioning clients for the court, must warn clients of their Fifth Amendment rights. By 1980 the Court (*Vitek v. Jones*, 445 U.S. 480 [1980]) described commitment as a "massive curtailment of liberty."

A second strand of new rights developed around the question of competence. A long-standing area of judicial review has focused on competency to stand trial. Over the post-1950 period, courts have increasingly examined the area of competency outside the criminal justice system. In most cases they have considered this question in relation to a person's ability to participate in treatment decisions, particularly when treatment is refused or forced medication is sought. The number of such cases that have appeared over the last twenty years is probably in large measure a result of the modern understanding that mental illness does not ipso facto equal mental incompetence or an inability to give informed consent (*Mills v. Rogers*, 457 U.S. 291 [1982]).

As public mental health systems and providers develop more innovative services and treatments for consumers, they face tensions between making mistakes that worsen the condition of people receiving mental health services and failing to make changes that will create substantially improved services or treatment possibilities. Where the state seeks to medicate or otherwise treat against the wishes of an individual, those tensions have often come before the courts for resolution.

The Supreme Court recognized some form of liberty interest in "avoiding the unwanted administration of antipsychotic drugs" in *Mills v. Rogers*. In remanding to the First Circuit Court of Appeals for further determinations, the Court commented that under Massachusetts law "an involuntary commitment provides no basis for an inference of legal 'incompetency.'" The Massachusetts Supreme Court subsequently found that in a nonemergency situation nothing justifies medication without a patient's permission and offered a definition of when forced medication is appropriate.

A final area of legal innovation has been the question of the right to appropriate treatment. In 1970 the *Wyatt v. Stickney* case commenced, challenging the conditions, treatment, and habilitation of the residents of one of Alabama's oldest institutions. The complaint behind this class action was originally brought by state employees. The case sought to establish a constitutional right to treatment, with such treatment being targeted to the reason for each person's confinement. Minimum standards were set in 1972 and a court monitor was appointed in 1977. What are known as Wyatt Standards both drive the development of community services and serve as the model for care in the hospital itself (see chapter 4).

Settlement agreements in other states have been based on intervention by the

U.S. Department of Justice (DOJ) under the Civil Rights of Institutionalized Persons Act (CRIPA).[3] The statute gives the DOJ the authority to investigate conditions in publicly operated facilities and to take action where there is a pattern or practice that deprives people in those facilities of their constitutional or federal statutory rights. Whereas older institutional cases relied on specific plaintiffs and classes of patients or residents, the DOJ can now respond to allegations of illegal conditions from patients, staff, relatives, the media, and Congress itself.

Most recently, the Court, in *Olmstead v. L.C. and E.W.* (119S.Ct. 2176 [1999]), held states accountable for placing persons with mental disabilities in community settings rather than institutions when the state's treatment professionals find community placement appropriate. It ruled that it is a form of discrimination under the Americans with Disabilities Act (ADA) for the state to fail to find community placements and unnecessarily keep individuals with disabilities in institutions. This case has been the impetus for renewed efforts to develop community-based services as alternatives to institutional care in some states. In others it has been a reason to reestablish the role of state institutions and to challenge Congress's right to impose ADA requirements on the states. Medicaid and other federal, state, and foundation resources have been directed to many of these efforts to create additional community-based services.

The significance of mental health law in the context of system change and the evolution of policy making is twofold. First, the courts have become important in policy making for mental health. Decisions by the courts have had far-reaching implications that have served to enhance consumerism and increase the costs of state hospital care, thereby precipitating the decline of those institutions, and have defined the boundary between the state's right to protect the public and the autonomy of individuals with the most severe mental disorders. The courts' second and indirect effect has been through their defining the choices open to psychiatric patients and the responsibilities of society to offer real therapeutic choices to patients. This has served to create a legal and regulatory environment that is strongly consistent with decentralized choices, consumerism, and the placement of purchasing power and decision making in the hands of people with mental disorders.

Contemporary Policy Making for Mental Health Care

Today's sources of policy advice and decision making regarding public resources aimed at caring for people who are mentally ill are a clear break from the first seventy years of the twentieth century. Since 1980 the National Association of State Mental Health Program Directors has tracked statistics on the mental health care resources under the control of state mental health agencies. Those data document the changing fortunes of the state mental health agencies in the United States. Nominal spending associated with state mental health agencies grew from $7.1 billion in 1981 to $9.3 billion in 1987 to $16.1 billion in 1997 to $20 billion in 2001. Table 6.1 shows state mental health agency spending in relation to total mental health spending and total spending on public mental health care. In all cases the state agency share has declined. The mental health agency share of public spending declined by about 15 percent from 1987 to 1997 and an additional 6.3 percent from 1997 to 2001. The share of the total declined by 10.3 percent from 1987 to 2001. This decline understates the reduction in the control of discretionary funds because state mental health spending is increasingly tied to Medicaid matching requirements as well as court-imposed legal requirements, which further reduce discretion in the use of state general fund dollars (Frank et al., 2003).

Within the states, the role of the state mental health agency has also declined as measured by their claims on resources. Since 1985 the share of state budgets accounted for by state mental health agencies fell from a high of 2.14 percent in 1983 to 1.81 percent in 1997 (Lutterman and Hogan, 2001). Mental health services and responsibility for people with mental illness are increasingly associated with other state agencies such as social welfare (e.g., foster care), the correctional system, juvenile justice, as well as the state Medicaid agency.

Moreover, the source of federal funds in the area in which state mental health agencies and mental health advocates have had the greatest discretion, the federal mental health block grant, has declined sharply as a share of state mental health spending. The decline in the block grant has contributed disproportionately to the decline in influence of mental health policy makers. The SAMHSA block

TABLE 6.1
*Funds Controlled by State Mental Health Agencies (SMHAs)
and Total Mental Health Spending*

	Billions of Dollars		
	1987	1997	2001
SMHAs	$ 9.3	$16.1	$20.0
Total public	$19.9	$40.5	$53.6
Total all sources	$35.7	$70.8	$85.4
SMHAs as % of public	46.7%	39.8%	37.3%
SMHAs as % of total	26.1%	22.7%	23.4%

SOURCES: Data from table 4.1 in this volume; NASMHPD Research
Institute, Funding sources and expenditures of state mental health agencies:
Fiscal year 2002 (www.nri-inc.org/RevExp/RE02/02Report.pdf).

grant has been the principal policy focus of advocacy groups (e.g., the National Alliance on Mental Illness), state mental health agency directors, and agencies that provide direct services. There is, in contrast, little representation of mental health interests at the advisory councils of the Social Security Administration (SSA), the Centers for Medicaid and Medicare Services (CMS), or the Department of Housing and Urban Development (HUD)—and these agencies are now much more important sources of mental health funding and policy making.[4]

Consumerism

At the turn of the twenty-first century, serious discussions of mental health care delivery and policy cannot be considered complete without a systematic assessment of consumerism in mental health care (US DHHS, CMHS, 1999; Salzer et al., 2001). Consumerism in mental health embodies a number of discrete activities. One has been the creation of self-help groups, which occurred primarily in the late 1980s and throughout the 1990s. Self-help programs include case-management programs, job coaching, social support, housing programs, and crisis services. These programs have served to fill gaps left by public and private organizations and to more closely tailor extant services to the needs and preferences of people with mental disorders. Many of the self-help programs are funded by state mental health agencies.

A second aspect of consumerism involves the organization of people with mental disorders and their families into effective political interest groups that aim to make specialty mental health providers and state mental health institutions more responsive to the people they serve. Federal agencies such as SAMHSA and the NIMH take careful account of the views of groups representing consumer interests through a range of mechanisms, from participation by consumer groups in advisory councils to consumer representation in the review of research grants at the NIMH. Consumer groups such as the National Alliance on Mental Illness (NAMI) have been enormously effective in increasing the level of funding for research on mental disorders at the NIMH and in influencing the research agenda.

The consumer movement in mental health generally focuses on enhancing the voice of consumers in the context of a centrally planned mental health delivery system (Salzer et al., 2001). Consumer groups rarely mention negotiating with the key social insurance institutions that today provide consumers with purchasing power. Consumer groups have, in fact, taken a less active role in improving the functioning of markets for mental health care through provision of education and information to consumers operating in a mental health delivery system that increasingly relies on markets to allocate resources. Their main thrust toward improved consumer decision making and more efficient markets for mental health has been in the area of case management. Case managers help to negotiate the patchwork of health insurance, social programs, and income support sources for people with severe mental disorders, which has become one of the great challenges for people with mental illness. Case managers, however, are typically employees of provider agencies, so their role in exercising consumer choice and promoting quality competition more broadly is quite limited.[5]

Organized mental health consumer interests have been far less involved in efforts to improve the quality and efficiency of health care delivery by creating more informed consumers and purchasers, although such activities have occurred. Because most people with disorders such as depression initially contact the general medical sector for care, one important development has been in improving the treatment of depression in primary care (Frank et al., 2003; Pincus, 2003). Some of the mechanisms used in this area have been the inclusion of quality indicators related to depression in consumer-oriented report cards and accreditation standards that aid purchasers in choosing among health plans.

The Role of Specialty Mental Health Policy Makers Today

Today the institutions that pay for care and support of people with mental disorders are private health insurance, Medicaid, Medicare, SSI/SSDI, Temporary Assistance to Needy Families (TANF), and other social service programs such as those run by HUD, the Department of Education, and the Department of Agriculture (food stamps). As a consequence, the public officials who traditionally exercised stewardship over mental health delivery wield less influence over the greatly expanded set of resources and policies that now treat and support people with mental disorders.

Modern policy entrepreneurs in the mental health system have in many cases been able to implement rather dramatic changes in the organization and financing of mental health care delivery. States such as Ohio, California, and Texas effected changes in the design of state mental health systems in the 1980s and 1990s that were far more sweeping in terms of structure and departure from traditional philosophies than were earlier changes.[6] Yet in most cases the effect of those dramatic initiatives was muted in comparison with that of the more modest changes of the earlier era. A basic reason for this was that the surrounding mainstream programs—Medicaid, Medicare, SSDI, SSI, and housing support programs—remained largely unchanged by these innovations.

The expansion of financial responsibility for mental health services and income support to different levels of government and to other parts of the bureaucracy within each level of government has fostered interest in treating people with mental illness like those with other medical conditions and in directly dealing with factors that set mental health care apart. Issues related to involuntary commitment, the special challenges of employment programs for people with severe mental disorders, and the influence of housing on treatment response by people with mental disorders all call for mental disorders to be handled in a special way.

These conflicting policy directions have tended to reinforce the distinction between the traditional mental health bureaucracy and new health and social insurance programs. Public mental health systems have become the bastions of mental health exceptionalism, whereas health and social programs have become places to "mainstream" mental health. The irony of this phenomenon is that mental health expertise and interest-group pressure remain concentrated on an ever-shrinking part of the resources devoted to care of mental illness in the United States.

The last decade of the twentieth century bore witness to a set of large health policy debates with profound implications for mental health care delivery that had very little systematic mental health policy input from either a technical or a political perspective. The debate around the Clinton health plan, the creation of the State Children's Health Insurance Program, Medicare prescription drug coverage, and plans to finance care for the uninsured all advocated endeavors with potentially profound effects on the well-being of people with mental illness. Rarely did these initiatives explicitly take account of the unique policy challenge posed by people with severe mental illnesses. This neglect has also been a feature of debate around critical social welfare programs, including Social Security's Ticket to Work program, welfare reform, and the Section 8 housing voucher programs (Rupp and Bell, 2003). People with mental disorders have benefited from the growth in resources that new programs have made available for their care, while the voice of the mental health community has steadily been muted by the slow adjustment to the shifting landscape of health and mental health policy.

Conclusions

The profound changes that have occurred over the past fifty years in the financing and supply of mental health services have invalidated the traditional structure of mental health policy making. State mental health authorities, historically the pillars of policy development and implementation, have been left controlling only a small fraction of mental health spending and an even smaller share of the supply of services. Instead, an array of mainstream programs and providers has captured an ever-growing share of this sector. This weakening of the institutional voice of mental health policy making leaves an important void, because mainstream program administrators rarely have the knowledge, or the need, to focus on the requirements of the population with mental illness. The same mismatch exists on the consumer side. The vibrant mental health consumer movement, originally organized to confront these same institutions, has a similarly limited voice as it seeks to address issues in mainstream programs. The ability to further improve the well-being of people with mental illness depends on the development of a policy and consumer voice for mental health care within the context of a range of mainstream programs.

CHAPTER 7

Assessing the Well-being of People with Mental Illness

Over the past five decades, Americans have witnessed vast improvements in living standards. Incomes have more than tripled (adjusting for inflation). The share of U.S. families living in poverty has fallen by half. The life expectancy of adults has increased seven years since 1950. Most Americans have benefited from a rich array of new treatments for life-threatening diseases, and they are better protected against the financial costs of those treatments. The quality of most of the other goods and services we purchase has also improved markedly. This chapter examines whether mental health delivery has kept pace with these developments and whether people with mental illnesses have shared in this generally rising tide of fortunes over the past fifty years.

As we have shown, the United States has invested heavily in treatment for mental disorders over the past five decades. There has been considerable innovation in the treatment of mental illnesses. By themselves, these investments and innovations would be expected to translate into improved well-being. At the same time, however, there have been profound changes in the nature of delivery of mental health services. Public mental hospitals have shrunk drastically. New private institutions, such as managed behavioral health organizations, have taken over many of the responsibilities of public mental health authorities. They have also replaced much of the private fee-for-service insurance system. Many observers have raised alarms that the development of new pharmacologic treatments has come at the cost of displacing other forms of therapy. Much of the popular discussion of the state of mental health suggests that the negative consequences of these institutional and therapeutic changes more than outweigh any gains from increased spending on services and innovation. In this chapter we will evaluate these conflicting claims through an assessment of the well-being of people with mental illness over time.

The ideal way to make such an assessment would be to study a comprehensive, longitudinal database. Using such data, we could examine whether, for example, Americans are better protected against the financial risks of mental illness, are receiving increasingly effective therapy, and are better supported in the event of a severe mental disorder. Unfortunately, no such single database exists. Instead, our strategy in making assessments over time is to combine information from multiple sources. Administrative data provide reasonably consistent information on the number of people served by the public mental health system in various settings. Epidemiologic surveys conducted at various times provide information on the number of people with specific types of mental illnesses. Numerous general health and medical surveys provide information on patterns of treatment and financing over time. Research studies offer assessments of the effectiveness of specific therapies.

We assembled these various sources of information to assess the availability and quality of treatment over the last five decades in a series of steps. First, we estimated the size of the population with mental illness and divided that population into categories that, in a particular context, are likely to be meaningfully different in terms of treatment and living arrangements. In assessing changes in the quality of treatment received, we divided the population of people with mental illness by major disorder category. Second, we used information from surveys conducted at different times to calculate the proportion of these populations that received any mental health treatment at all. Third, we further subdivided the population according to the type of treatment received. For example, we used information from health care surveys to measure the share of people with depression who were receiving an antidepressant at each of several points. Fourth, we used the most recently available information from research studies to project the likely effect of a particular type of treatment on a person with a particular disorder. These data are rarely rich enough to permit a precise measurement of effectiveness. Rather, we divided treatments received into broad quality categories—likely to be highly effective, likely to be somewhat effective, no evidence of effectiveness, and likely to be harmful. We then extrapolated the probable effectiveness of observed patterns of treatment in the past on the basis of our understanding of treatment today.

We used a similar process to assess changes in living conditions. We divided the population by the severity of their functional disabilities. We then focused mainly on those with severe mental illness. We identified and classified the living situations in which people with mental illness can be found. We collected information from administrative sources and surveys to estimate how many people are located in each of the relevant settings. For example, data exist on the number of people who are residents of psychiatric institutions or who are homeless at various points. These data do not, however, generally indicate what proportion of the population that is located in a particular setting is severely mentally ill. Furthermore, that proportion is likely to have changed over time. Data from current studies and from prior reports are used to estimate these proportions. Combining these data, we constructed estimates of the proportion of people with mental illness who are in each type of setting. Finally, we collected data on the economic circumstances of people found in each setting.

Treatment

For people with mental illness, the receipt of treatment that reduces the disabling consequences of illness is likely to be a central component of well-being. As we documented in chapter 3, the technologies available to treat mental illness have changed over time. In the years before 1950, better treatment of infectious disease had nearly eliminated some important causes of mental illness, chiefly syphilitic brain disorder. Treatments developed in the postwar period also offered the first routinely effective therapies for the symptoms of schizophrenia and major depression. Although these new treatment technologies developed after 1960 only occasionally have surpassed earlier modalities in terms of their efficacy in controlled clinical trials, many of them are easier for providers to administer and simpler for patients to take and tolerate. The result has been improved adherence to recommended treatment and, hence, improved outcome. In some other areas, such as the treatment of anxiety disorders, new pharmacologic agents represent a more significant advance in the efficacy of treatment, along with improved tolerability and reduced risk of addiction. The proliferation of effective treatments within each category also means that the potential for matching patients to treatments has improved.

Since the 1950s the supply of providers of mental health services has increased notably. Both the total number of professionals and provider institutions and the range of professionals and institutions have expanded. This increase in supply, too, should improve access to services and offer greater choice of treatment strategy.

Finally, financing policy over this period has helped people with severe mental illness gain access to services outside psychiatric institutions. Because services are financed through an insurance model, rather than providers being funded directly, people with mental illness have been given more autonomy in selecting the type of treatment and setting for their care. The increased breadth of insurance (and the absence of a fixed budget) has also resulted in expanded financial protection for all insured Americans against the consequences of mental illness. This expanded coverage, however, provides no assistance for people who lack health insurance altogether.

We examined two aspects of treatment over time: the receipt of any treatment and the quality of treatment received.

Does Increased Receipt of Treatment Reflect an Improvement in Well-being?

A primary goal of mental health policy since 1950 has been to provide effective treatment to people with mental illness. Correspondingly, we argue that evidence that more people are receiving better treatment provides one piece of evidence that the well-being of people with mental illness has improved. There are several potential objections to this approach.

The value of treating mental illness—however effectively—has been continually challenged. An enduring theme in the development of civil rights for people with mental illness is the question of when people have a right to refuse treatment. To the extent that treatment is not received voluntarily, increases in prevalence of treatment cannot be viewed as necessarily improving well-being. In 1997 fewer than 5 percent of persons in treatment for a mental illness were referred to care by a court (Sinaiko and McGuire, 2005). In 1980, 28.7 percent of specialty psychiatric admissions were involuntarily (US DHHS, 1985). In 1994 nearly 43 percent of days of specialty inpatient psychiatric care were accounted for by people involuntarily admitted; this statistic reflects a roughly similar number of admissions, though the majority of these admissions did not pass through the courts (Frank and McGuire, 2000). Only 4 percent of admissions in 1980 were involuntary and related to criminal activity. Even among those not involuntarily committed, some may have felt other pressures to accept treatment (Monahan et al., 2003). Another vocal but tiny minority of researchers has argued that even fully voluntary treatment—particularly medication treatment—of mental illness is inappropriate. In this view, mental illness is a social construct that describes behavior society views as deviant. Such behavior should be accommodated, not masked by treatment. This ideological position had its greatest popular currency in the 1960s. The belief that treatment is not a suitable response to mental illness, however, continues to play a part in public debate around, for example, the treatment of social phobia and ADHD in children (NIH Consensus Statement, 1998). As we have shown, improvements in the effectiveness of treatment vary across the range of disorders, from those where effectiveness is not well established (borderline personality disorder) to those, such as major depression, where the value of effective treatment is based on strong evidence.

Finally, even if treatment is appropriate, critics argue, it is frequently inappropriately applied in specific cases. This type of misallocation has been widely documented in other areas of medical practice, such as heart bypass surgery, and there is ample evidence that such misallocation happens in mental health as well. A particularly clever statement of misallocation in mental health care in the 1950s came from the renowned psychiatrist Jerome Frank (1961): "The pattern of psychotherapeutic practice in America is seriously imbalanced in that too many of the ablest, most experienced psychiatrists spend most of their time with patients who need them least."

Practitioners often disagree about indicators for treatment, which leads to divergences in practices. In our analysis we often relied on utilization data that provided little, if any, information about whether treatment was appropriate. We found, however, that there is some evidence of improvements in the match between condition and treatment over time.

Receipt of Any Treatment

We collected information on the proportion of the population with mental illness who received any treatment for their condition from epidemiologic community surveys, public opinion surveys, three national surveys of health care expenditures and financing, and ongoing surveys of ambulatory medical care. These measures serve as indicators of changing access to mental health services. Unfortunately, indicators of the receipt of services do not provide any information on the quality of services that may have been received. We will examine the quality of care separately later in this chapter.

PROVIDER-BASED DATA

For the period since 1977, we examined data on office visits to physicians for outpatient services through the National Center for Health Statistics' National Ambulatory Medical Care Surveys (NAMCS). These data show an increase over time in the percentage of visits to physicians at which a mental health diagnosis was recorded (fig. 7.1). This increase is composed of two elements. First, there has been a sea change in the nature of psychiatrists' office practice. In 1977, 64 percent of psychiatrist visits consisted of psychotherapy only, without medications prescribed or continued. By 2002 the fraction of such visits had fallen to

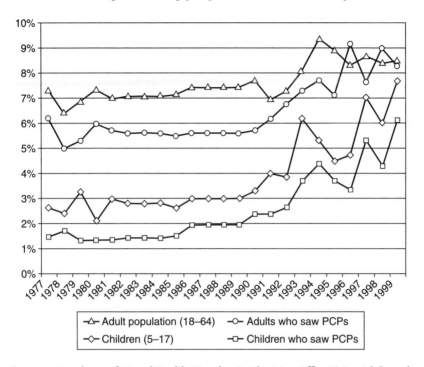

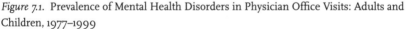

Figure 7.1. Prevalence of Mental Health Disorders in Physician Office Visits: Adults and Children, 1977–1999

SOURCE: Data from National Ambulatory Medical Care Survey (1977, 1978, 1979, 1980, 1981, 1985, 1989, 1990–2000).

10 percent; almost all psychiatrist visits by this time incorporated medications and these visits were typically much shorter than therapy-only visits. In consequence, although the total number of psychiatrists increased by only 11 percent over this period, the total number of visits to psychiatrists increased by 34 percent (authors' analyses of the National Center for Health Statistics, NAMCS, and US DHHS, 2003, 292, table 100).

Second, primary care physicians (PCPs) now play a more active role in mental health treatment. We do not have good data on the treatment of mental health in primary care before 1977. In 1977 just 6 percent of visits to a primary care physician recorded treatment of a mental health problem. By the late 1990s this figure had increased to more than 8 percent. Almost all this increase occurred after 1992. This pattern is even stronger among children. Primary care treatment rates for mental disorders began climbing in 1990 and have continued to increase steadily since then.[1]

One concern about this finding is that general practitioners might have treated patients without recording a psychiatric diagnosis. Our data do not support this hypothesis—we observed little change in the share of patients seen by PCPs who had psychiatric symptoms but did not receive a psychiatric diagnosis.[2]

We do not have consistent provider-based data for nonphysician providers. Population data, however, provide information on the full range of provider types.

POPULATION-BASED DATA

The first source of population-based data is information from epidemiologic surveys. Figure 7.2 presents available information on treatment prevalence rates for mental illness from such surveys. These surveys (discussed in detail in chapter 2) used different methods to estimate prevalence and count different types of services as treatment. Some (such as the Epidemiologic Catchment Area study [ECA] and the National Comorbidity Survey [NCS]) examined the share of a population that reported using mental health services of some type. Others (such as the Baltimore, New Haven, and midtown Manhattan studies) counted the institutionalized population and divided by the relevant denominator population. These studies suggest an enormous increase in outpatient specialty mental health treatment between the midtown Manhattan study and the ECA, followed by a smaller increase between the ECA and NCS studies. By 2001 the NCS replicate study showed that the percentage of the population receiving any treatment for a mental health problem grew to 20.1 percent from 12.2 percent in 1991. Among people with a disorder in a given year, the rate of treatment in 2001 was 41.1 percent, compared to 20.3 percent in 1991, a large increase (Kessler et al., 2005).

A second source of information is social survey data. Kulka, Veroff, and Douvan (1979) examined the rate of mental health services in two waves of data (1957 and 1976) collected on social attitudes by the Institute of Social Research at the University of Michigan. They reported that overall service use for mental health problems rose from 14 percent in 1957 to 26 percent in 1976. In both years, however, much of this consisted of nonformal mental health services (e.g., clergy, lawyers, and others). They found that 2 percent of respondents had ever used a psychiatrist's or psychologist's services in the 1957 survey, whereas 7 percent had done so in the 1976 survey. By contrast, in the 1991 NCS 17 percent of respondents reported ever having seen a psychiatrist or psychologist, and 32 percent reported ever having sought professional services (including general physician or counselor services) for a mental or emotional problem. This comparison again suggests a very large increase in service use between the mid-1970s and 1990.

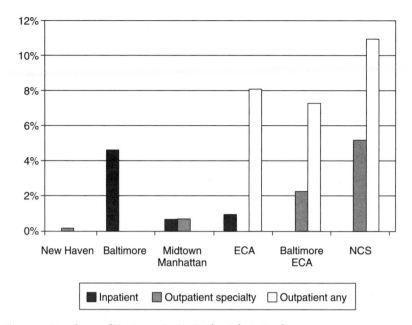

Figure 7.2. Prevalence of Treatment in Six Epidemiologic Studies

SOURCES: Data for New Haven (1958) from Hollingshead and Redlich, 1958. Data for Baltimore Community (1957) from Pasamanick, 1957, 1962. Data for Midtown Manhattan (1962) from Srole et al., 1962. Data for ECA (1980) from Robins and Regier, 1980. Data for NCS from Kessler et al., 1994. Data for Baltimore ECA (1981–84) from Eaton et al., 1997.

Finally, we turn to information from surveys of health service use. We compare the use of health services in a given year for a *diagnosed* mental health condition across three national surveys: the National Medical Care Expenditure Survey (NMCES; 1977), the National Medical Expenditure Survey (NMES; 1987), and the Medical Expenditure Panel Survey (MEPS; 1996) (table 7.1). Adult use of services over this period shows a slightly declining rate of diagnosed and treated prevalence between 1977 (5.2%) and 1987 (4.8%), followed by a 60 percent increase in treatment prevalence rates, to 7.7 percent, between 1987 and 1996 (percentage treated for a diagnosed mental disorder). Although these data suggest a considerably lower prevalence of treatment rate than the 11 percent in the NCS of 1991, people without a current diagnosis accounted for about 33 percent of the NCS number. Counting only cases with both treatment and diagnosis (to make the figures comparable to the MEPS data), prevalence of treatment in the NCS is 7.3 percent. In the second row of the table, we adjusted these figures to reflect the estimated prevalence of illness in the community. These figures suggest that the proportion of people with a diagnosable disorder who received formal mental

TABLE 7.I.
Treated Prevalence Rate, All Psychiatric Disorders

	NMCES 1977	NMES 1987	MEPS 1996
Percentage of all adults 18–64 with a mental health diagnosis at a treatment visit	5.2	4.8	7.7
Estimated percentage of all adults with a mental health disorder receiving treatment[a]	17.6	16.6	25.7

[a]Based on prevalence of treatment estimated from National Medical Care Expenditure Survey (NMCES, 1977), National Medical Expenditure Survey (NMES, 1987), and Medical Expenditure Panel Survey (MEPS, 1996) and estimated epidemiologic prevalence from chapter 2.

health treatment has never exceeded 30 percent, but that the fraction has been increasing since 1987.

PREVALENCE OF TREATMENT IN THE GENERAL POPULATION

The data show marked increases in treatment rates over this period, although, as we noted in chapter 2, there is little evidence of an increase in the underlying prevalence of disorder over time. Prevalence of treatment appears to have increased particularly rapidly over two periods, 1957–76 and 1987–2000. Our evidence about patterns in prevalence of treatment during the 1976–87 period is more mixed: the proportion of the population reporting ever having used mental health specialty services increased substantially, but the rate of prevalence of mental health problems diagnosed at visits remained flat.[3]

WHY DID THE RATE OF TREATMENT INCREASE?

One reason for increasing treatment rates has been the expansion of health insurance coverage over this period. We do not have direct evidence of the role of expanded coverage before 1977. Over the 1977–96 period rates of treatment increased for both insured and uninsured people, but they increased more for those with coverage. People with no coverage were 24 percent more likely to be treated in 1996 than in 1977. The privately insured population was 50 percent more likely to obtain mental health care in 1996 than it was in 1977. About 7.5 percent of people with private insurance received treatment for a mental disorder in 1996, up from 5 percent in 1977. The largest increase in rates of treatment was for people with Medicare or Medicaid coverage, a 68 percent rise. In part this is a consequence of changes in the characteristics of the population with this type of coverage over this period. During the 1980s and 1990s a growing fraction of

Medicaid and Medicare beneficiaries became eligible for public insurance because of a disability related to a mental illness (Stapleton et al., 1998).

The pattern of sharply increasing treatment rates among privately insured persons since the late 1980s is striking because this period coincided with the growth of managed behavioral health care. Managed behavioral health care organizations ration care directly. The rise of this alternative form of rationing has generally led to reductions in the out-of-pocket costs of service. Our findings suggest that this new pattern of rationing has increased rather than reduced the fraction of the population receiving services.

A second reason for the increase in treatment has been changes in treatment technologies. The availability of new drug therapies has made it easier for physicians to treat prevalent mental disorders such as depression and anxiety. Information about drugs such as Prozac may have encouraged more people with symptoms of mental disorders to obtain care. In addition, private insurance coverage for prescription drugs expanded rapidly during the late 1980s and early 1990s.

We found that among those with mental health diagnoses who saw office-based physicians, treatments involving psychotropic drugs accounted for nearly all the growth in prevalence of treatment between 1977 and 1996, which is consistent with the development of these new therapies. At the same time, however, we found that treatment rates for people for whom drugs were not prescribed was nearly constant over the 1977–96 interval. This pattern suggests that the introduction of new psychotropic drugs primarily expanded the total population receiving treatment, rather than substituting for other forms of therapy. This is consistent with the notion that expansion of health insurance coupled with the availability of new user-friendly treatments made treatment more accessible and attractive.

PREVALENCE OF TREATMENT AMONG THOSE WITH SEVERE AND PERSISTENT MENTAL ILLNESS

The pattern of changes in prevalence of treatment is somewhat different for those who are seriously and persistently mentally ill. Our denominator for these analyses is the population prevalence of serious and persistent mental illness (SPMI). Data from 1955 suggest that most treatment episodes occurred in inpatient settings. We assume that 50 percent of people with SPMI who were not in hospitals received treatment, a very generous estimate reflecting the prevalence of treatment among inpatients (Hollingshead and Redlich, 1958). We assume that beginning in the mid-1960s, 80 percent of nonhospitalized SPMI patients received treatment, a figure that is consistent with studies done in 1978 and 1989, which suggest that it did not change much over the last forty years (US PCMH, 1978a; Talbott, 1978; Barker et al., 1992).

We used information from hospital studies and staffing information to estimate the fraction of patients in state hospitals who were receiving treatment beyond custodial care at various points. In the 1950s studies suggest that between 50 percent and 66 percent of hospitalized patients received any treatment beyond custodial care, most at low intensity (Hollingshead and Redlich, 1958; Redlich and Kellert, 1978). Over the succeeding fifty years, staffing ratios in inpatient institutions climbed rapidly. By 1976 professional staff per bed in state and county hospitals were double the 1950 figure. Ten years later staffing had more than doubled again. Staffing remained stable at 1986 levels through the 1990s. On the basis of these staffing changes, we assumed that at least 80 percent of hospitalized patients were receiving regular treatment by the mid-1970s, and that 100 percent were receiving treatment after 1986.

The evidence of increased staffing levels in psychiatric hospitals over the period of deinstitutionalization has a surprising implication for prevalence of treatment among people with SPMI. We found that it remained relatively stable and may even have increased at various times through most of the period of deinstitutionalization. Even though public psychiatric hospital systems were shrinking, treatment intensity for those who remained in hospitals was rising, which offset the relatively lower probability of receiving treatment in the community. By the mid-1970s treatment intensity in institutions was quite high and, in the same period, most—though not all—people with SPMI outside institutions reported receiving some treatment.

Quality of Treatment Received

More people have been receiving treatment over time. But what has happened to the quality of that treatment? Information about this issue is available only sporadically and from scattered and inconsistent sources. Early studies of treatment patterns rarely related treatment to current diagnostic definitions, and so it is especially difficult to assess the match between condition and treatment.

We gathered evidence on the effectiveness of different forms of mental health treatment primarily from guideline and consensus panels that have been conducted by the NIMH, the American Psychiatric Association (APA), and the schizophrenia Patient Outcomes Research Team (PORT). As we noted in chapter 3, current consensus panels do not provide information on treatments that have fallen out of favor. We searched for the most recent available information about treatments that had been mentioned over time and added this information to the consensus panel data. We placed treatments in four categories of effectiveness. Table 7.2 shows our classification of current and historical treatments for these diagnoses.

The final column in table 7.2 lists treatments that have been shown to be harmful. One of the most notable improvements in mental health care in the early part of this period was a reduction in the use of these therapies. Among psychiatric patients hospitalized in the 1950s who received any treatment, more than 66 percent received electroconvulsive therapy, insulin shock therapy, or lobotomies. As late as 1973, more than four hundred psychosurgeries were performed on average each year. Use of electroconvulsive therapy declined substantially between the mid-1970s and the late 1980s.

The best data to evaluate the evolution of treatment quality are available for the treatment of depression (table 7.3). The earliest data, from the mid-1970s, show that even among hospitalized patients with depression, only 17 percent were receiving therapy now judged likely to be highly effective. This fraction varied over time but did not rise above 40 percent until the mid-1990s. By the mid-1990s roughly half of outpatient cases of depression were receiving treatments that were likely to be highly effective (Busch, Berndt, and Frank, 2001). By the latter 1990s, McGlynn et al. (2003) estimated that on average people with depression in private health plans received 57 percent of recommended appropriate treatment.

Table 7.4 repeats this analysis for the treatment of schizophrenia. Many early treatments for schizophrenia were, in retrospect, harmful to patients. Early advances consisted of eliminating these treatments. Gradually, treatment improved, but as late as 1980 nearly 33 percent of patients with a diagnosis of schizophrenia

TABLE 7.2
Categories of Treatment Efficacy

	Likely to Be Highly Effective	Likely to Be Somewhat Effective	No Evidence of Effectiveness	Likely to Be Harmful
Major depression	SSRIs and TCAs Cognitive behavioral therapy/ interpersonal therapy	Electroconvulsive therapy (psychotic and severe) MAOIs	Psychodynamic psychotherapy Tranquilizers/ sleeping pills	Electroconvulsive therapy (under certain conditions)
Schizophrenia	Chlorpromazine Supportive counseling in combination with drugs	Assertive community therapy/ cognitive behavioral therapy	Psychodynamic psychotherapies Hydrotherapy	Insulin shock therapy Psychosurgery Electroconvulsive therapy

SOURCE: Based on analyses of treatment evolution and treatment guidelines in chapter 3.

TABLE 7.3
Quality and Prevalence of Treatment of Major Depression, 1975–1997

1975–76[a]	Likely to be highly effective Antidepressant: 17.2%
	Likely to be somewhat effective Minor tranquilizer: 34.5% Sleeping pill: 17.2%
1978–80[b]	Likely to be highly effective 200+ mg of imipramine for four consecutive weeks: 49% of inpatients, 19% of outpatients
	Likely to be somewhat effective Neuroleptic: 19% of inpatients, 3% of outpatients Anxiolytic: 36% of inpatients, 24% of outpatients Lithium carbonate: 6% of inpatients, 1% of outpatients
	Unclear efficacy Electroconvulsive therapy (ECT) (depending on type of depression/conditions of use, but no evidence of effectiveness at best): 19% of inpatients Psychotherapy (depending on type): 95% of inpatients received any psychotherapy, 57% received an hour or more per week; 97% of outpatients received some, 48% received an hour or more per week
1982[c]	Likely to be highly effective 150+ mg of antidepressant or MAOI: 12%
	Likely to be somewhat effective 1–150 mg of antidepressant or MAOI: 23% Neuroleptic: 25% Minor tranquilizer: 55% Lithium carbonate: 4% ECT: 21% of psychotic depressed, 8% of severely depressed
	Unclear efficacy ECT (depending on conditions, but no evidence of effectiveness at best): for neurotic depression: nonpsychotics > 4/wk 6%; nonpsychotic > 12/wk 6%; nonpsychotic > 26/wk 9%; suicidal behavior, nonpsychotic 10% Psychotherapy (depending on type and length): 67%
1987[d]	Likely to be highly effective Antidepressant (non-SSRI): 37.3%
	Likely to be somewhat effective Anxiolytic: 15.7% Antipsychotic: 4.6% Mood stabilizer: 3.1% Stimulant: 0.1%
	Unclear efficacy Psychotherapy (depending on type and length): 71.1%
1997[d]	Likely to be highly effective Antidepressant (SSRI): 58.3% Antidepressant (other): 28%
	Likely to be somewhat effective Anxiolytic: 13.1% Antipsychotic: 3.6% Mood stabilizer: 8.8% Stimulant: 0.7%
	Unclear efficacy Psychotherapy (depending on type and length): 60.2%

[a]Weissman et al., 1981. [b]Keller et al., 1986. [c]Keller et al., 1982. [d]Olfson et al., 2002.

TABLE 7.4
Quality and Prevalence of Treatment of Schizophrenia, 1940–1996

1940–46[a]	Likely to be harmful or ineffective	Electroconvulsive therapy (ECT) or insulin shock therapy: 100%
Late 1950s[b]	Likely to be somewhat effective	Directive psychotherapy or drug therapy (unspecified): 23%
	Likely to be harmful	Insulin shock or psychosurgery: 20%
	Unclear efficacy	Nondirective psychotherapies, ECT, and unspecified organic therapies (unknown prevalence)
1975[c]	Likely to be effective	Drug therapy: 25%
	Not likely to be effective	Individual psychotherapy: 25%
1996[d]	Likely to be very effective	Drug therapy (following PORT guidelines): 40+%

[a] Joint Commission on Mental Illness and Health, 1961.
[b] Hollingshead and Redlich, 1958.
[c] Redlich and Kellert, 1978.
[d] Lehman and Steinwachs, 1998.

who were seeing an office-based physician for treatment on an outpatient basis received only psychotherapy, a treatment that was unlikely to be efficacious (authors' analyses of the NAMCS). By the late 1990s this figure had fallen below 5 percent. We have no information about the quality of prescribing practices in the earlier period, but because later studies suggest that many patients still do not receive appropriate doses of antipsychotic medications, it is probable that many of those receiving antipsychotic medications were not receiving an adequate dose.

In the mid-1990s the schizophrenia PORT project reviewed patterns of care for patients with schizophrenia. The criteria used were far more stringent than those applied in the earlier surveys and, in many ways, the results were quite disappointing. Nonetheless, in comparison with earlier years, the PORT documented substantial improvements in the quality of treatment: more than 40 percent of patients received appropriate treatment on most dimensions. Data from Florida Medicaid for the period of 1994–2000 offers a mixed picture of quality of care for schizophrenia (Frank et al., 2004). Use of antipsychotic agents continued to increase and reached 90 percent in 2000. The use of newer atypical antipsychotic agents by people with schizophrenia rose from 19 percent in 1994 to 61 percent in 2000. In contrast, use of individual and group therapy or counseling declined from 52 percent in 1994 to 30 percent in 2000. Similarly, psychosocial rehabilitation care use fell from about 50 percent of Medicaid beneficiaries with schizophrenia to 40 percent over the 1994–2000 period.

We also examined treatment patterns for patients with anxiety disorders. Here we have data only on medication treatment and cannot document changes in the rate of use of efficacious psychotherapies. There were steady increases between 1977 and 2000 in the percentage of patients with a diagnosis of anxiety disorder who were treated with medications. Among them we observed a pronounced switch to newer, more efficacious agents, such as SSRIs, from the earlier benzodiazepines (e.g., Valium and Librium) and, by the end of this period, the complete exnovation of Miltown, an agent with significant negative side effects (authors' analyses of the NAMCS). These patterns are consistent with our findings for depression and schizophrenia, which implies improvements in the quality of treatment provided to patients with anxiety disorders.

Recent analyses of the usual care of privately insured people with bipolar disorder shows that the use of recommended components of treatment remained stable during the first half of the 1990s, that the intensity of care has increased, and that the amount of inappropriate care has declined (Ling et al., 2004). Thus, by 1995, 63 percent of people treated for bipolar disorder in private plans were being treated with mood stabilizers, and 83 percent were getting psychotherapy. Among those receiving psychotherapy the number of visits per user increased from 1991 to 1995. Finally, the portion of patients receiving clearly inappropriate care declined from 7.7 to 5.9 percent (ibid.).

Many patients receiving care have illnesses other than depression, schizophrenia, anxiety, or bipolar disorder. We have no information on changes in the quality of treatment for these conditions. In some cases, efficacious treatments for them have not yet been identified. In others, there is no consistent historical record that would allow us to make comparisons.

Our data are also very weak in describing changes in the quality of psychotherapeutic interventions received. Data on the quality of psychotherapy are not now and never have been available. The use of experimentally validated therapies remains the exception in treatment today. Nonetheless, the expanding array of validated therapies suggests that their use is probably increasing.

Our results suggest that the rate of receipt of quality mental health treatment has improved over the past fifty years. The prevalence of receipt of any treatment for a mental disorder has been rising for the population as a whole and has at least held steady for the seriously ill population (Mechanic and Bilder, 2004; Kessler et al., 2005). The quality of treatment received has shown consistent improvements for both groups, as receipt of ineffective and harmful treatment has fallen and receipt of treatment likely to prove effective has risen.

These improvements have occurred even though, in most cases, the treatments available for alleviating symptoms of key mental illnesses (depression and schizophrenia) are not much more efficacious than those that existed in the mid-1960s. Rather, improvements in the ease of prescribing and using treatments have extended the reach of effective treatments to a greater share of the population.

The Financial Burden of Illness

People with mental illness continue to pay a larger share of their expenditures out of pocket than do those with other serious illnesses. Insurance coverage for mental health care has never been as complete as that for other serious health conditions. Yet financial protection against the costs of mental illness has also improved over time. Out-of-pocket spending has declined markedly as a share of total mental health care spending since 1971, falling from nearly 35 percent to about 17 percent in 1997 (Levine and Levine, 1975; Coffey et al., 2000).

Data on out-of-pocket payments at the individual level are available for the period since 1977 from the NMCES, NMES, and MEPS. Out-of-pocket payments for mental health services among adults with mental illness were relatively stable between 1977 and 1987 and fell somewhat between 1987 and 1996 (table 7.5). In 1977, 23 percent of spending for mental health care was paid for out of pocket. In 1987, 24 percent of mental health spending was paid for out of pocket. Comparable figures from the MEPS suggest a reduction in the out-of-pocket share since 1987 to below the 1977 level. Note that the real out-of-pocket spending level has increased since 1977 because total expenditures on mental health have increased.

Improvements in financial protection took two forms: expansions in insurance coverage and changes in the content of insurance.

Insurance Coverage

The most important change in financial protection over this period was the introduction of the Medicaid program, which gave people with serious mental illness who were not hospitalized a source of financing for their care. Since its enactment in 1965, Medicaid has become increasingly valuable to people with SPMI. An increasing number of people with SPMI are also eligible for Medicare. Medicare disability insurance became available to disabled people who qualify for Social Security Disability Insurance (SSDI) beginning in 1972. Many disabled people with Medicare are also eligible for Medicaid because their income is sufficiently low. We estimate that in 2001 some 1.3 million persons with a SPMI had Medicare coverage.

In 1972 Medicaid covered about 24 percent of the population with SPMI, whereas

TABLE 7.5
Per Capita Spending on Mental Health Services for Adults with Psychiatric Disorders

	1977 (N=1,106)		1987 (N=847)		1996 (N=927)	
	1996 $	% OOP[a]	1996 $	% OOP	1996 $	% OOP
All mental health	759	23	1,539	24	1,185	21
Physician visits	209	28	386	40	276	30
Nonphysician visits	29	56	140	54	108	34
Prescriptions	55	68	124	51	339	34
Hospital admissions	446	12	715	8	417	3
Outpatient visits	13	17	158	14	31	6
Emergency	7	27	16	10	14	11

SOURCES: Data from National Medical Care Expenditure Survey (1977), National Medical Expenditure Survey (1987), and Medical Expenditure Panel Survey (1996).
[a] Percentage of total spent out of pocket.

by 1998 we estimate that Medicare and Medicaid covered more than 60 percent of this population. Likewise, McAlpine and Mechanic (2000) used the health care community survey to estimate that 80 percent of people whom they classify as having a severe mental illness had some insurance coverage in 1998. Our estimate of Medicare coverage, while high, is also roughly consistent with information from hospital discharge surveys. In 1979 about 19 percent of inpatient discharges with a primary diagnosis of schizophrenia were paid for by Medicare (authors' analyses of the National Hospital Discharge Survey). By 1999 about 50 percent were paid by Medicare.

Mental health insurance coverage also expanded for those in the general population. Few private insurance plans today exclude coverage for mental illness, although this was common practice before the 1970s. Nonetheless, people with mental health diagnoses remain more likely to be uninsured than the population generally (McAlpine and Mechanic, 2000). In 1998 community surveys, the share of people with a diagnosable mental illness who were uninsured was 20.4 percent for people with a severe mental illness (SMI) and 18.2 percent for those with a non-SMI diagnosis of a mental disorder; 11.4 percent of people with no disorder were uninsured (ibid.).

Expanded Financial Protection within Insurance

The results above for the population as a whole hold for both publicly and privately insured individuals. For privately insured people, mental health expenditures increased from 1977 to 1987 and fell from 1987 to 1996 to a level that remained more than 50 percent above the 1977 level. The share of expenditures paid out of pocket fell steadily from 29 percent to 22 percent. For publicly insured people, the pattern was similar, with the 1996 level about one-third above the 1977 level. The share of expenditures paid out of pocket was consistently much lower for this group, but it rose over this period from 1 percent to 7 percent of total mental health expenditures. By contrast, there was little change in mental health expenditures from 1977 to 1996 among uninsured people, and the share they paid out of pocket increased from 29 percent to 50 percent.[4]

Consumers of mental health services are considerably better protected against the cost of care today than in earlier years. These improvements have come about because of general expansions of the scope and reach of insurance coverage, including the introduction of coverage for prescription drug expenditures. At the same time, the introduction of managed care techniques has reduced reliance on the use of cost sharing to ration care in the health insurance market. This picture is not entirely unclouded, however; many people with mental illness are uninsured and lack access to useful services.

Work

The ability to participate in the labor market is tremendously important to people with mental illness. Work offers both income and a connection to society. Thus, changes in the ability to work over time provide a good indicator of living circumstances, particularly for people with less severe mental illness.

We have little information on changes in labor force participation among people with mental illness in the past. Changes in the nature of work, from jobs that relied mainly on physical strength toward those requiring more education, may have disadvantaged people with mental illnesses. By contrast, improvements in treatment technologies and in the prevalence of treatment have meant that a smaller proportion of those affected by mental illness now experience prolonged disabling symptoms (Berndt et al., 2002). Passage of the Americans with Disabilities Act in 1990 expanded the statutory rights of people with mental illness to participate in the labor market.

The evidence on the ability of people to obtain and hold jobs suggests that the effect of mental disorders on employment has remained quite stable—and consistently poor—when their employment is compared to that of the general population. For example, Bartel and Taubman (1979, 1986) studied a cohort of male veterans in the 1970s and found that having a diagnosed mental disorder reduced employment levels by 6.8 percent. Ettner, Frank, and Kessler (1997) used data from the National Comorbidity Survey and found that a diagnosable mental disorder reduced employment among men by between 8 and 12 percent. Similarly, the effect of mental disorders on earnings has also remained relatively consistent across studies over time. Bartel and Taubman (1986) estimated a decrease in earnings attributable to mental illness of about 25 percent. Frank and Gertler (1991) used data from the ECA survey and estimated a 21 percent reduction in earning for men that was associated with mental illness. Ettner, Frank, and Kessler (1997) estimated a somewhat smaller effect of a mental disorder on males using the 1991 National Comorbidity data, although they considered a somewhat broader set of disorders. They found reductions in male earnings ranging from 12 to 21 percent (depending on the estimation method).

A number of studies have examined the influence of severe mental illnesses on work. Mechanic, Bilder, and McAlpine (2002) examined four large surveys and reported that 22 to 40 percent of people with schizophrenia worked in the 1990s and only 12 percent worked full-time. This compares to adult employment rates of 75 percent to 83 percent overall. The comparable rates of employment for the larger category of people with severe mental illness were 32 percent to 61 percent. Yellin and Cisternas (1996) examined rates of employment for people disabled by mental disorders compared to rates for people with other types of disabling conditions for the years 1982–91. They reported that people disabled by mental illnesses consistently had the lowest rates of labor-force participation. People disabled by mental illnesses worked at roughly 50 percent of the rate of people with other disabling conditions. Finally, Salkever (2003) found that people with psychiatric disabilities who obtain jobs are less likely to retain their jobs than are people with other types of disabilities. Thus, the effect of severe mental disorders on work appears to be large and consistent over time.

Living Conditions

Social insurance plays a critical long-run role in assuring that basic human needs are met for people with SPMI. Although new treatments enable many people with mental illness to recover from some of the effects of their disorders, significant numbers of people with mental illness, even if receiving appropriate treatment, continue to experience substantial functional impairment as a consequence of their illnesses. For this group, public policy has a critical role to play in ensuring the adequacy of living conditions.

We examined three aspects of living conditions for people with SPMI: living arrangements, resources, and legal rights.

Living Arrangements

Several studies have examined factors affecting the satisfaction with quality of life of people with SPMI. That research shows that people with mental illness, like most Americans, prefer living circumstances that offer them privacy and give them contact with their families and with social support. Most studies find that people are more satisfied with life in the community than in the hospital.[5]

Using these studies, we created a simple preference ordering for living arrangements among people with SPMI. We inferred that situations that permit people with mental illnesses to live independently or with their families are most preferred, whereas situations in which people are homeless or incarcerated are least preferred. Other settings fall somewhere between these extremes, but we do not rank them.

To assess the living circumstances of people with SPMI, we extrapolated from limited information on different living situations. Many studies examine the fraction of people in a particular type of living situation who have a mental illness. Using these proportions, information about the total number of people living in each situation, and our estimate of the size of the population with SPMI, we then calculated the share of the SPMI population who live in each of these settings.

Table 7.6 shows that the living arrangements for the adult population with SPMI have changed dramatically over time. In 1950 psychiatric hospitals housed about 494,000 people between the ages of eighteen and sixty-four. Among this group, we estimated (on the basis of Kramer's 1977 tabulations) that about 27 percent had organic brain disorders, including senility, which would not be included in our SPMI definition today. This leaves a total of 361,000 SPMI people aged eighteen to sixty-four living in psychiatric institutions at that time. That is, nonelderly adults with SPMI accounted for less than three-fourths of the total population of these institutions in 1950. We estimated that an additional 93,000 people with SPMI in this age group lived in other institutional settings, including nursing homes.

The living situations of elderly people with SPMI have also changed. Most have moved out of psychiatric institutions and into nursing homes, a phenomenon known as transinstitutionalization. It is unclear whether this transition has benefited or harmed them.

The very limited data available suggest that rates of incarceration of people with SPMI (as a fraction of all those incarcerated) have remained relatively stable over time, so the share of SPMI people incarcerated varies principally with the overall incarceration rate. We estimated that about 18,000 people aged eighteen to sixty-four with SPMI were incarcerated in 1950, when jail and prison populations were much smaller than today.

The homeless population was also much smaller in 1950 than at present, and some research suggests that the prevalence of mental illness among homeless adults has increased over time. We estimated that in 1960 some 23,000 people with SPMI were homeless.

Contrary to much popular perception, a majority of people with SPMI did not live in institutions even in 1950. We estimated that more than 10 percent lived with their families. Many others lived in boardinghouses, flophouses, or hotels. Living conditions in these settings were probably very poor, but some privacy was available.

Combining this information, we estimated that 2–3 percent of the SPMI population lived primarily in the least desirable settings (homeless or incarcerated) in 1950, 30 percent were institutionalized in psychiatric hospitals, nursing homes, or other institutions, and about 60 percent lived with family or in other settings ("Other/Unknown" in table 7.6).

It is clear that by 1970 the living arrangements of people with mental illness had changed substantially. In 1970 only 15 percent of people aged eighteen to sixty-four with SPMI lived in psychiatric institutions, and an additional 7 percent lived in nursing homes or other institutional settings. Though institutionalization had declined, neither incarceration nor homelessness had increased very much. We estimated that about 2 percent of people with SPMI continued to live in the very worst circumstances (incarcerated or homeless).

By 1990 psychiatric hospitals, nursing homes, and other institutions housed a very small share of the population with SPMI—less than 10 percent at any point. Many people with SPMI were affected by the general rise in incarceration and in homelessness. We estimated that about 3 percent of the SPMI population was incarcerated and about 3 percent were homeless, which means that twice as many people were in poor living circumstances as had been the case in earlier decades. Notably, however, we observed an increase in the share of people living with family members and independently. We estimated that more than 80 percent of people with SPMI were housed in the community by 1990.

Incarceration rates rose further between 1990 and 2000, leading to a greater increase in the share of the population with SPMI who were in jail or prison. Despite this increase, the proportion of people living with family or in the community remained roughly stable over the decade of the 1990s.

The patterns described above suggest that most, though not all, people with

TABLE 7.6
Living Arrangements of People with Severe and Persistent Mental Illness, Ages 18–64
(in Thousands)

	1950	1960	1970	1980	1990	2000
Number with SPMI[a] in all living arrangements	1,570	1,700	1,960	2,350	2,620	2,890
Noninstitutionalized						
Total noninstitutionalized with SPMI		295	222	205	320	430
SPMI noninstitutionalized, as percentage of all SPMI		17%	11%	9%	12%	15%
Living with family[b]						
Number disabled and living with family		618	586	608	893	1,066
Percentage with SPMI		27%	27%	27%	30%	35%
Number with SPMI		167	158	164	268	373
SPMI living with family, as percentage of all SPMI		10%	8%	7%	11%	13%
Board and care[c]						
Number in board and care					96	219
Percentage with SPMI					26%	26%
Number with SPMI					25	57
SPMI in board and care, as percentage of all SPMI					1%	2%
Hotels and boardinghouses[c]						
Number in hotels and boardinghouses		642	320	204	137	
Percentage with SPMI		20%	20%	20%	20%	
Number with SPMI		128	64	41	27	
SPMI in hotels and boardinghouses, as percentage of all SPMI		8%	3%	2%	1%	

NOTE: Ages are 18–64 unless other ages are noted.

[a] We assumed that 17 people per 1,000 have serious and persistent mental illness (SPMI). This is about 50% above the average of the rates found by Ashbaugh et al. (1983), Barker et al. (1992), the Urban Institute (as reported in Talbott [1978]), and the U.S. Department of Health and Human Services (1980).

[b] We estimated the number living with family from the decennial census. We took the number of adults aged 25–55 who are out of the labor force and living in a household where the head of the house is a parent, stepparent, or other family member. We assumed that 50% of men and 40% of women living with their parents, and 30% of women living with another relative, had a disability (based on the 1990 and 2000 census, where these data were available). Among this disabled population, we assumed that 27% had a serious and persistent mental illness in 1960, 1970, and 1980, 30% in 1990, and 35% in 2000 (from the rates of mental illness among the SSI disabled population [US SSA, 2001]).

[c] Hotel and boardinghouse population data are from the census, as reported in Jencks (1994). We assumed that 20% of hotel and boardinghouse occupants had SPMI (Burt, 1992). For board and care occupants, we estimated the number aged 18–64 from the 1990 and 2000 census. The census does not use the terminology "board and care facility," but the definition of "group home" most closely matches that of board and care facilities (Clark et al., 1994). We excluded those in drug rehabilitation homes and those in homes for unwed mothers. The 2000 census shows that 61% of noninstitutionalized group quarters individuals, excluding military personnel and college students, were 18–64. We used this rate for both the 1990 and the 2000 numbers. We assumed that 26% of nonelderly residents of adult group homes are mentally ill. This number is from the 1991 National Health Provider Inventory survey. Of the 22–64-year-old group home residents in that survey, 26% were in a group home that was primarily responsible for treating people with mental illness.

(continues)

TABLE 7.6 *(continued)*

	1950	1960	1970	1980	1990	2000
Institutionalized in Health Care Facilities[d]						
Total SPMI institutionalized in health care facilities	454		433		237	170
SPMI institutionalized in health care facilities, as percentage of all SPMI	29%		22%		9%	7%
Mental institutions						
Number in mental institutions	494		351		103	54
Percentage without organic brain disorder or senility	73%		86%		94%	94%
Number without organic brain disorder or senility	361		302		97	51
SPMI in mental institutions without organic brain disorder or senility, as percentage of all SPMI	23%		15%		4%	2%
Nursing homes						
Number in nursing homes	28		81		169	163
Percentage with SPMI	46%		46%		46%	46%
Number with SPMI	13		37		79	75
SPMI in nursing homes, as percentage of all SPMI	1%		2%		3%	3%
Other health care facilities						
Number in other nonjuvenile health care facilities	159		188		123	88
Percentage with SPMI	50%		50%		50%	50%
Number with SPMI	80		95		62	44
SPMI in other nonjuvenile health care facilities, as percentage of all SPMI	5%		5%		2%	2%
Other Institutionalized[d]						
Total SPMI in other institutions	20		26		83	144
SPMI in other institutions, as percentage of all SPMI	1%		1%		3%	5%

[d]The total number of people in institutions is from the census, Persons in Group Quarters (US BC, 1990). The 1990 and 2000 figures are from the census Web site, and the 1950 and 1970 numbers are reported in U.S. President's Commission on Mental Health (1978a). The category "other health care facilities" includes homes for the mentally handicapped, chronic disease hospitals, and any other institution the census included in its count. To get the population aged 18–64: in 2000, the data were broken down by age group. We assumed for nursing homes, "other health care facilities," and juvenile institutions that the same proportion of these populations was 18–64 for all years. For correctional institutions, we assumed that 99% of the population was in this age group in 1950, 1970, and 1990 (O'Flaherty, 1996). For mental institutions, we assumed that 80% of the population was in this age group in 1950, 1970, and 1990, as this is the percentage reported in the 1986 Client/Patient Sample Survey (Rosenstein, 1990). For nursing homes, we assumed that 46% of the population was SPMI (Kessler et al., 1998). This percentage may be a bit high, but as there is a very small percentage of nursing home patients aged 18–64, it should have a negligible effect on our results. For juvenile institutions and "other health care facilities," we also followed Kessler et al. (ibid.) in assuming that 50% of residents had SPMI. For mental institutions, we assumed that 100% of the population aged 18–64 was seriously and persistently mentally ill (ibid.). For correctional institutions, we used Diamond et al. (2001) in assuming that 7% of inmates aged 18–64 had SPMI.

TABLE 7.6 *(continued)*

	1950	1960	1970	1980	1990	2000
Other Institutionalized[d]						
Correctional institutions						
Number in correctional institutions	264		326		1,103	1,938
Percentage with SPMI	7%		7%		7%	7%
Number with SPMI	18		23		77	136
SPMI in correctional institutions, as percentage of all SPMI	1%		1%		3%	5%
Juvenile institutions						
Number in juvenile institutions who are 18 or older	5		7		12	15
Percentage with SPMI	50%		50%		50%	50%
Number with SPMI	2		3		6	8
SPMI among those 18 or older in juvenile institutions, as percentage of all SPMI	0.1%		0.2%		0.2%	0.3%
Homeless[e]						
Number of homeless		113		121	262	228
Percentage with SPMI		20%		20%	30%	30%
Number with SPMI		23		24	79	68
SPMI who are homeless, as percentage of all SPMI		1%		1%	3%	2%
Other/Unknown[f]						
SPMI whose living arrangements are unaccounted for in this table, as percentage of all SPMI	51%	55%	65%	72%	73%	71%

[e] We estimated the population between 18–64 that is homeless from the rates reported in Jencks (1994, 17, table 2). This gave us rates for 1980 and 1990. For 1960 we used the 1958 Chicago study estimates (Jencks, 1994) and assumed that Chicago was representative of nationwide trends. For 2000 we used the 1996 estimate published by the Urban Institute that 444,000 people are homeless at one time. We assumed that 20% of the homeless in 1980 and earlier and 30% after 1980 were SPMI (Burt, 1992).

[f] This category was obtained by subtracting all the categories of SPMI living arrangements from the total population aged 18–64 with SPMI. For people living with their families, we assumed that the 1950 rate was the same as in 1960. For the hotels and boardinghouses, we assumed that the 1950 rate was the same as the 1960 rate and that the 2000 rate was the same as the 1990 rate. For persons in institutions in 1960 and 1980, we assumed that the rates were halfway between those for 1950 and 1970 and 1970 and 1990, respectively. Likewise, for the homeless, we assumed that the rate in 1950 equaled the rate in 1960 and the rate in 1970 was halfway between those for 1960 and 1980.

mental illness live in circumstances at least as good today as at most times over the past fifty years. Some, however, clearly live in much poorer circumstances —homeless or incarcerated. Our data suggest that it would be a mistake to attribute the increase in homelessness and incarceration among people with SPMI directly to the experience of deinstitutionalization. Increases in homelessness and incarceration are, for the most part, associated with increases in the proportion of the entire population (most of whom do not have SPMI) who experience these undesirable circumstances. Increases in the overall homelessness rate have been attributed to changes in the low-income housing market that affected all people—including many noninstitutionalized people with SPMI—who relied on these markets (O'Flaherty, 1996). Likewise, increases in incarceration rates due to the war on drugs and crackdowns on quality-of-life crimes (community policing) would have affected both those deinstitutionalized and the many people with SPMI who would not have been living in institutions even if deinstitutionalization had not taken place.

Resources

Individual well-being depends not only on living arrangements, but also on the resources available to support them. We now examine the resources available to people with SPMI in institutions and outside them over time.

The resources available to institutions serving people with SPMI increased dramatically over the last half of the twentieth century. The level of staffing per bed in public psychiatric hospitals more than quadrupled and expenditures per bed also increased. To put these increases in expenditures into context, we compared per bed expenditures with the federal poverty line (FPL). Across all psychiatric institutions, expenditures per bed increased approximately fivefold compared to the FPL between 1970 and 1994 (from 3.3 times to 15.1 times the FPL). Another way of measuring the resource intensity of institutional care is to compare it to the cost of living outside institutions. We created an artificial basic resource bundle, consisting of the per capita value of SSI, Medicaid, assisted housing, and food stamps. By the late 1990s expenditures per bed in mental institutions were approximately eight times higher than the corresponding monetary value of the basic resource bundle. By contrast, before the mid-1960s, the value of the basic resource bundle (adjusted for inflation) was greater than the expenditure per bed. It is important to note that the severity of illness and other problems associated with the institutional population has also increased.

Table 7.7 shows that resources available to people with mental illness outside institutions have also shown nearly continuous improvement. The average annual value of Medicaid benefits has nearly tripled (from about $3,400 to $9,600), and the fraction of people receiving Medicaid has increased. The fraction receiving Medicare benefits also increased in the late 1990s. Medicare spent about $3.23 billion on people under age sixty-five with SPMI (Foote and Hogan, 2001). About half of those with Medicare were also eligible for Medicaid.

The implementation of SSI and SSDI substantially increased the resources available to disabled people living in the community and often replaced the inconsistent general assistance benefits that had previously been provided by states and localities. With the exception of the early 1980s, the proportion of people with SPMI receiving SSI has increased more or less continuously since the inception of the program. In 1980 approximately 24 percent of the severely mentally ill adult population received SSI payments, whereas in 1998 about 41 percent received these benefits. Sincer 1985 the average SSI award for a disabled individual has stayed more or less constant at just over 50 percent of the FPL for an individual under age sixty-five. The federally mandated SSI amount per individual has remained at about 70 percent of the FPL; however, many disabled people do not receive the full amount because other sources of income, including SSDI, are counted against this total.

We estimated that in 1980 about 11 percent of people with SPMI were covered by SSDI; by 2000 the number was approximately 30 percent. The rate of receipt of SSDI benefits has increased rapidly since the inception of the program, with a particularly sharp increase since 1990 (which may be attributable to more generous benefits; Autor and Duggan, 2003). We report the average benefit received for all beneficiaries because data on benefits by diagnosis type are limited. In 2001, however, the average benefit received by those with a mental disorder was $737 per month, just slightly less than the average for all disorders ($772). Real benefits per recipient increased substantially between 1965 and 1980 and have remained flat since, at about 100 percent of the FPL. Taken together, SSDI and SSI expanded support for people with SPMI between 1986 and 2002. People receiving SSI, and others with low incomes, also receive in-kind aid from the government, the most common form of which is food stamps. The proportion of SPMI people who receive food stamps has risen: food stamps were introduced in 1961, national eligibility levels were established in 1971, and then eligibility for the program was expanded. The average annual value of food stamp benefits has more than doubled, from $419 to $904.

Housing assistance is one of the most valuable benefits for people with mental illness. The principal available form of housing assistance is a Section 8 housing

TABLE 7.7
Ingredients of Improved Living Conditions

	1960	1965	1972	1974	1980	1990	1998
Number of adults (18–64) with SPMI (in millions)[a]	1.70	1.81	2.03	2.11	2.35	2.62	2.89
Food stamps (enacted in 1961)[b]							
Percentage of SPMI receiving food stamps		1%	31%	35%	52%	47%	63%
Average annual value of food stamps benefit		$419	$666	$738	$861	$935	$904
Medicaid (enacted in 1965, linked to SSI in 1972)[c]							
Percentage of SPMI receiving Medicaid			24%	33%	35%	39%	60%
Average annual value of Medicaid benefit			$3,400	$4,100	$5,600	$8,700	$9,600
Medicare (linked to SSDI in 1974)[d]							
Percentage of SPMI receiving Medicare				9%	11%	24%	32%
Average annual value of Medicare benefit				$1,900	$3,200	$4,600	$5,500
SSI (enacted in 1972/benefits 1974)[e]							
Percentage of SPMI receiving SSI				23%	24%	30%	41%
Average annual SSI award for disabled				$5,015	$4,789	$4,844	$4,893
Federal allotted SSI payment (individual in own household)				$6,060	$5,969	$6,114	$6,284
SSDI (enacted in 1956)[f]							
Percentage of SPMI receiving SSDI		25%	7%	9%	11%	22%	30%
Average annual SSDI payment		$6,417	$8,866	$8,615	$9,297	$9,301	$9,325
Section 8 housing (enacted in 1974)[g]							
Percentage of SPMI receiving incremental voucher					0.2%	0.2%	0.0%
Percentage of SPMI receiving cumulative voucher					2.2%	3.9%	4.1%
Average HUD outlay per assisted renter					$3,265	$3,940	$4,500

[a] Total number of people aged 18–64 is from the Council of Economic Advisers, 2002. Because the report uses a 16–19-year-old age group, we assumed that half of the 16–19-year-olds are 18 or 19. We assumed that 17 people per 1,000 have serious and persistent mental illness. This is about 50% above the average of the rates found by Ashbaugh et al. (1983), Barker et al. (1992), the Urban Institute (as reported in Talbott [1978]), and the U.S. Department of Health and Human Services (1980).

[b] The total number of people receiving food stamps is from US SSA (2001). We then found the percentage of food stamp recipients who also received SSI from House Committee on Ways and Means (2004), table 15-10. Data were available only beginning in 1980. We assumed that the 1980 rate held for earlier data. We assumed that 32% of adult SSI recipients have SPMI (Long et al., 2002). The average annual value of food stamps is from US SSA (2001). We multiplied the average monthly value by twelve and inflated the numbers to 2000 dollars.

[c] The total number of people receiving Medicaid is from US SSA (2001). We included just the people receiving Medicaid because of total or permanent disability. We assumed that the share of this population between 18 and 64 is the same as the percentage of those receiving SSI in this age group (as reported ibid.) We assumed that 32% of adult Medicaid total or permanent disability recipients have mental illness (see note e below). We used the value of Medicaid benefits for recipients with permanent and total disability from US SSA (2001) and inflation-adjusted to 2000 dollars. The 1974 estimate uses 1975 data.

[d] The total number of people receiving Medicare is listed in House Committee on Ways and Means (2000). We used the people receiving Medicare because of disability. We assumed that the share of Medicare total or permanent disability recipients who had mental illness follows that for SSDI (see note f below). We used the average value of Medicare benefits in US SSA (2001). The 1974 estimate uses 1975 data.

[e] All data are from US SSA (2001). We assume that 32% of recipients aged 18–64 are SPMI, an average of data from 1987, 1989, 1991–93, 1995, and 1997–2000 (the only available years). The average annual value of an SSI payment is from ibid. We took the average value for disabled recipients and inflated to 2000 dollars. The 1974 value estimate is actually from 1975.

[f] The total number of disabled workers is from US SSA (2001). We then took (from ibid.) the percentage of these with a mental disorder and the fraction of new awards for mental disorders for various years. We used linear interpolation to estimate the figure for 1965, 1974, and 1980. The average annual benefit to disabled workers is also from ibid.

[g] The total number of incremental and cumulative housing vouchers is from US DHUD (2000). We used the total number of vouchers or certificates. We assumed that 84% of Section 8 recipients are 18–64 (as reported on the HUD Web site). We assumed that 10% of adult recipients are SPMI. This is based on several reported statistics (US DHUD, 1990, 1993, 1995). We calculated the average HUD outlay per assisted renter using data reported in Quigley (1999). We inflated to 2000 dollars. The 1980 incremental number is actually from 1981.

voucher. The Section 8 voucher program, enacted in 1974, provides very valuable benefits, but few people receive this assistance. In total, Section 8 has provided housing vouchers to approximately 4 percent of the SPMI population, most of which were distributed during the 1980s. The average outlay per assisted renter from the U.S. Department Housing and Urban Development has increased from about $3,265 per year in 1980 to $4,500 in 1998.

Housing conditions in general have also improved between 1950 and 2000. The percent of people living in "cage hotels" (in which rooms are divided only by wire fencing), flophouses, YMCAs, hotel rooms, and boardinghouses has declined dramatically (Jencks, 1994). The condition of housing units has improved. For example, the number of one-room apartments with incomplete plumbing fell by 93 percent between 1960 and 1990 (ibid.). The number of "crowded apartments" (apartments with more than one person per room) has fallen from 20 percent of apartments in 1940 to 3 percent in 2000. And the number of severely crowded apartments (more than one and a half persons per room) has fallen from 9 percent to under 3 percent.

The broad expansion of financial support that became available to people with mental illness, particularly since the mid-1970s, has resulted in unambiguous improvement in the lives of the significant fraction of people with SPMI who live outside institutions. Though public insurance programs provide benefits that rarely suffice to lift people out of poverty, they do provide more reliable support than the patchwork of programs that preceded them. Few of these programs were specifically directed at people with mental illness. Yet the expansion of income support programs has been extraordinarily valuable to people with SPMI, empowering them to make basic choices about living arrangements and sometimes allowing them to exercise greater choice among mental health service providers.

Rights

By most measures, changes to the legal system over the last fifty years have improved the well-being of people with SPMI. People are entitled to treatment and if civilly committed must have treatment related to the purpose of their commitment. People cannot be medicated for the convenience of staff. Patients cannot be used as an unpaid labor force. People with SPMI who are concerned about many of the side effects of psychiatric medications can in some circumstances refuse treatment.

Between 1966 and the end of the 1970s, the principles of equal protection (due process) and equal treatment (education and minimum wage, e.g.) were formally extended to people with mental illness. Since then, these rights have been extended and formalized. By 1985 the Supreme Court had declared that zoning laws cannot prevent people with mental illness from living in certain areas (*Cleburne v. Cleburne Living Center, Inc.,* 473 U.S. 432 [1985]). Unnecessary use of restraints and seclusion has resulted in civil settlements, although the monetary awards have not been large (*Ihler v. Chisolm,* 995 F. 2d 439, no. 98-712 [2000]). Finally, by 2002 twelve states recognized advance directives for psychiatric treatment as a mechanism for specifying preferred and unacceptable treatments (Bazelon Center, 2002).

In June 1999 the Supreme Court issued the *Olmstead* decision, a ruling that institutionalization of persons capable of receiving community-based treatment constitutes discrimination. The ruling recognizes that an institution may be the only appropriate care setting for some individuals, but it requires states to make community-based alternatives available to those who might benefit from them.

In summary, though quality of life is an elusive concept to measure, it appears to have improved for the adult population with SPMI. Many with severe mental illness have left institutional settings and are now, for the most part, in settings that are at least as good, if not better. There are now, both inside and outside institutions, more resources available, and those resources are of an increasing quality. Though a significant minority of people are worse off—incarcerated or homeless, rather than living in other institutions—most people with SPMI have more options and better living conditions today than they did during the past fifty years.

Stigma

One final aspect of the well-being of people with mental illnesses is the attitude of others in the community toward them. Negative views of persons with mental illnesses, or stigma, lead others to avoid living, socializing, or working with, renting to, or employing people with mental illnesses (Borinstein, 1992).[6] Although we have documented extensive changes in social policies, court decisions, treatments, and living conditions, we have found surprisingly little evidence of significant shifts in public perceptions about mental illness.

We focused on four key dimensions of the public's views: the way the public defines mental illness, views on the causes of psychiatric disorders, the level of avoidance of people with mental illnesses, and the perceived link between mental illnesses and violence. We examined public opinion surveys and conducted content analyses of media coverage of mental illnesses. The wording of questions in public opinion surveys has changed significantly over time.[7] Moreover, the

TABLE 7.8

Definitions of Mental Illness: Categorized Responses to an Open-ended Question

Diagnostic Categories with Which Respondents' Descriptions of Mental Illness Corresponded	Star's Survey 1950 (N = 337)	General Social Survey 1996 (N = 653)
Psychosis	40.7%	34.9%*
Anxiety or depression	48.7%	34.3%**
Social deviance	7.1%	15.5%**
Mental deficiency or cognitive impairment	6.5%	13.8%**
Other nonpsychotic disorder	7.1%	20.1%**

SOURCE: Data from Star (1950); GSS, 1996; Phelan et al., 2000.
NOTE: The question asked was "When you hear someone say that a person is 'mentally ill,' what does that mean to you?" Up to three categories were coded per respondent, so percentages exceed 100.
*p <0.10; **p<0.001 (two-tailed tests).

population samples used in most of the older opinion surveys were not nationally representative. Thus, the primary data set on which we relied is the Mental Health Module of the 1996 General Social Survey (GSS), which repeated questions asked in older surveys, particularly the pathbreaking work of Shirley Star in the 1950s.[8] We supplemented public opinion data with information on mass media coverage of mental heath and mental illness.[9]

The Definition of Mental Illness

Between 1950 and 1996 the public's definition of mental illness broadened (Phelan et al., 2000). In 1950 the vast majority of Americans defined mental illness as psychosis, anxiety, or depression. By 1996 a number of people also described behavior consistent with social deviance, mental deficiency, and other nonpsychotic syndromes, which suggests a more nuanced view of mental illness (table 7.8).[10]

This broadening of the public's definition of mental illness is consistent with the finding that the number of specific mental disorders discussed in popular magazines increased between the mid-1960s and the late 1980s, as did the number of stories on mental health topics in popular periodicals in general (Wahl and Kaye, 1992). Whereas articles in the 1960s discussed mental illness and "insanity" in broad terms, by 1988 articles were focused on distinct diagnoses, including attention deficit disorder and borderline personality disorder. Both the public's broader definition of mental illness and the trend toward increased media coverage of specific disorders are consistent with the general thrust of changes to the *Diagnostic and Statistical Manual* over time (Phelan et al., 2000).

Causes of Mental Illness

Although no earlier public opinion surveys elicited views on the causes of mental illnesses, the 1996 GSS suggested a more refined, multicausal view of mental illnesses than Star's pessimistic characterization of the public's views in the 1950s suggested (Star, 1955; Link et al., 1999). The 1996 GSS found that most Americans embrace the view that the causes of mental illnesses are multifaceted and vary across illnesses. The survey asked about six potential causes of alcohol dependence, major depression, schizophrenia, cocaine dependence, and being a "troubled person." A substantial number pointed to "stressful circumstances" as a cause of all these conditions. The extent to which other causes were attributed varied across illnesses (table 7.9). For instance, respondents were much more likely to say that a "chemical imbalance in the brain" was the cause of schizophrenia (84.6% saying somewhat or very likely) than of cocaine addition (48.2% saying somewhat or very likely).

Analyses of media content also suggested changes in views of causes of mental illnesses. For instance, an analysis of media coverage of schizophrenia found that between 1964 and 1992 the number of articles that linked schizophrenia to poor parenting dropped dramatically. By 1980 more articles explicitly stated that parenting style was not the cause of schizophrenia than implicated parents in children's illnesses (Wahl et al., 1995). Likewise, stories in more recent years have tended to focus on a range of causes, including heredity and biochemical dysfunction.

Avoidance of Persons with Mental Illness

Despite their broader views of mental illness and its causes, people are no more willing to have social connections with people with mental illness today than in the past. In the 1960s, 28 percent of individuals from a community sample in New York said that it is unwise to encourage a close friendship with someone who had been in a mental hospital (Dohrenwend and Chin-Shong, 1967). Roughly two-thirds (62.7%) agreed that one should discourage one's children from marrying someone who had been in a mental hospital. The 1996 GSS solicited preferences for social interaction with people described as having drug or alcohol dependency, schizophrenia, or depression. More than one-third (38.2%) of respondents reported being unwilling to befriend a person having these mental health problems. Nearly seven of ten (68.4%) said they were unwilling to have someone with drug or alcohol dependency, schizophrenia, or depression

TABLE 7.9
Perceived Causes of Selected Conditions

Perceived Cause	Alcohol Dependence[a]	Major Depressive Disorder[b]	Schizophrenia[c]	Cocaine Dependence[d]	Troubled Person[e]
The person's own bad character	51.3%	38.2%	32.8%	66.1%	39.9%
Chemical imbalance in the brain	62.8	72.8	84.6	48.2	42.8
The way the person was raised	65.9	47.6	45.1	41.7	58.0
Stressful circumstances in the person's life	91.9	94.8	90.7	72.0	93.5
Genetic or inherited problem	60.2	52.9	67.0	27.3	38.1
God's will	9.0	15.4	17.4	5.6	27.6

SOURCES: Data from GSS, 1996; Link et al., 1999.
NOTE: Percentages represent "very likely" and "somewhat likely" responses.
[a]Alcohol tolerance, withdrawal symptoms, inability to cut down or control use, change in functioning.
[b]Depressed mood, loss of interest and pleasure, insomnia, fatigue, feelings of worthlessness, inability to concentrate, social withdrawal.
[c]Delusions, auditory hallucinations, social and occupational impairment.
[d]Withdrawal symptoms, inability to stop use, occupational impairment.
[e]Subclinical mild worrying, sadness, nervousness, sleep problems, with no functional impairment.

marry a family member (Martin, Pescosolido, and Tuch, 2000). Though important methodological differences between these two surveys make comparison difficult, these data indicate that the desire to maintain social distance from people with mental illnesses remains significant.

Mental Illness and Violence

A major contributor to the negative views surrounding mental illnesses is the perception of a link between mental illnesses and violent behavior. Between 1950 and 1996 the number of people who mentioned violent or other types of frightening behavior in their definitions of mental illness nearly doubled to more than 12 percent (table 7.10). The increase was mainly among people who defined mental illnesses in terms of psychosis. Of that group, 31 percent mentioned violent or disturbing behavior in 1996, compared to only 13 percent of those who included psychosis in their definition in 1950 (Phelan et al., 2000).

TABLE 7.10
*Perceptions of Link between Mental Illness and Violence:
Categorized Responses to an Open-ended Question*

Perceptions of Violence and Other Frightening Characteristics	Star's Survey 1950 (N = 337)	General Social Survey 1996 (N = 653)
Percentage of respondents mentioning violent symptoms or manifestations	7.2%	12.1%*
Percentage of respondents whose descriptions were classified as "violent psychosis"	6.8%	12.4%**
Mean number of mentions of other frightening characteristics (extreme or excessive, unstable, unpredictable, uncontrolled, irrational)	0.23	0.31*

SOURCE: Data from Phelan et al., 2000.
NOTE: The question asked was "When you hear someone say that a person is 'mentally ill,' what does that mean to you?"
*$p < 0.05$; **$p < 0.01$ (two-tailed tests).

Longitudinal studies have not shown an increase in the frequency of stories or programs that contain violent and mentally ill characters. For instance, there was no increase in the number of characters in prime-time network television dramas who were mentally ill and violent between 1969 and 1985 (Signorielli, 1989), nor was there an increase in the number of stories connecting mental illness with violence in major newspapers between 1989 and 1994 (Wahl, 1996).

Opinion surveys suggest that the public holds a broader yet in some ways more stigmatized view of mental illness now than it did in the 1950s. On the one hand, Americans' definitions of mental illness include more types of disorders, and the public is less likely to attribute mental illness to personal weakness or parental influence than in the 1950s. On the other hand, a substantial number of people still want to limit contact with people with mental illnesses, and the number of people who mentioned violent behavior in their descriptions of mental illnesses nearly doubled between 1950 and 1996.

Conclusions

Across a broad array of dimensions, people with mental illness are doing better today than in the past. More people are receiving treatment; the available effective treatment alternatives have expanded, thereby improving the chances of finding a good match between patient and treatment. This potential seems to be realized in part in rising levels of use of recommended treatments. Financial protection and civil rights have improved. For some, treatment permits participation in the workforce. For those who are too disabled to work, the social safety net has been reinforced over time.

Improved treatment for mental illness, a growing supply of mental health professionals, and enhanced private insurance coverage have contributed to greater use of services by those with less serious conditions. There has been a startling increase in the fraction of this population who are receiving treatment—effective treatment—for conditions that would have gone untreated in the past. The rise in pharmacotherapy has supplemented, not displaced, a wide array of other services.

The civil and legal rights of people with mental illness increased nearly continuously over this period. Broader rights, expanded resources, and more accessible treatments reinforced one another to generate improvements in the lives of people with mental illness. Interestingly, all these mechanisms occurred despite a lack of improvement in public attitudes toward people with mental illness. This apparent contradiction illustrates the power of mainstream programs to improve the condition of people with mental illness. Mainstream programs and legal arguments built on broad concepts of rights could reach this population despite the continuing stigma attached to people with mental illness.

For the publicly insured, much of the improvement has been a consequence of public policy. The introduction of mainstream health insurance and social insurance programs has disproportionately benefited the most disadvantaged groups in society, particularly those with mental illness. By tying money to individuals rather than to providers or programs, these mainstream programs provide financial autonomy that buttresses the civil rights of people with mental illness.

Despite these successes, the situation of people with mental illness today is hardly desirable. Many people do not receive appropriate or adequate treatment. It remains difficult for people with mental illness to succeed in the workplace. Financial protections against the cost of illness are still less adequate for mental illness than for other types of illness. And mainstream social programs provide benefits that are insufficient to lift a single adult even up to the poverty line.

The lessons of the past suggest directions for much-needed further improvements. Innovation needs to focus on treatments that are not only efficacious but also readily disseminated into practice. Innovation in these directions is most likely to reach those who need it. Alternative forms of rationing, such as managed care techniques, are clearly effective in limiting excessive use of services. Substitution of such strategies for financial rationing through cost sharing will further expand access to treatment. Finally, increasing the level of benefits in programs for the disabled is an essential element of improving their well-being.

Such expansions come at a cost: they are likely to increase the number of people who participate in disability insurance programs. Here, too, more intensive management that limits inappropriate access may be an effective strategy. Even without it, society is better off erring on the side of generosity as it considers how to treat a severely disabled population.

CHAPTER 8

Looking Forward

Improving the Well-being of People with Mental Illness

In 1963 President Kennedy set out a "to-do list" for improving the quality of mental health care in the United States and the lives of people with mental disorders:

> We must act to bestow the full benefits of our society to those who suffer from mental disabilities; to prevent occurrence of mental illness . . . wherever and whenever possible; to provide for early diagnosis and continuous care in the community, of those suffering from these disorders; to stimulate improvements in the level of care given the mentally disabled in our State and private institutions, and to reorient those programs to a community-centered approach; to reduce, over a number of years and by hundreds of thousands, the persons confined to these institutions; to retain in and return to, the community population with mental illness . . . and there to restore and revitalize their lives through better health programs and strengthened educational and rehabilitation services. (Kennedy, 1963)

From the vantage point of the year 2006, it looks as though the United States took President Kennedy's vision seriously. The nation has made notable progress toward nearly all the goals he articulated in 1963. The lives of people with mental disorders are much more similar to those of most Americans today than they were in 1960. The material lives of the majority of people with these conditions are measurably improved. Their chances of clinical recovery and of regaining or maintaining the ability to function in society are greater now than ever in the past. Today people with severe mental disorders share more completely in the freedoms offered by U.S. society than they did in 1950, 1960, or 1970. Americans with mental disorders now have claims on material resources and human rights that simply did not exist thirty years ago.

The path taken to these outcomes has differed remarkably from the vision offered by President Kennedy and by advisors such as Robert Felix (1965). Their vision was of a mental health care system led by specialty mental health professionals and by institutions such as community mental health centers (CMHCs), built on the therapeutic advances of the 1950s and early 1960s.

The forces that actually drove the field were quite different. Technical advances in psychopharmacology and to a lesser extent psychotherapy did drive therapeutic gains in the period after 1965, but these gains involved increased "user-friendliness," not the improved therapeutic efficacy that the architects of community mental health care expected. Innovations in the financing and delivery of community-based care originated not in specialty mental health care, but in mainstream social insurance. The enactment of Medicare and Medicaid in 1965 gave most people with severe mental illnesses the ability to purchase a relatively rich array of clinical services in the community. The initiation of Supplemental Security Income (SSI) and Social Security Disability Insurance (SSDI) provided sources of income support to people disabled by a mental disorder that made it possible for them to buy food, obtain housing, and pay for other goods and services. Together, these policies gave people the ability to subsist in the community.

This difference between the vision and its realization sheds light on the ongoing tension between calls for mental health exceptionalism and calls to "mainstream" the care and support of people with mental illnesses. The dynamics of mental health care during the latter half of the twentieth century reflected these currents of thought. Mental health exceptionalism has been invoked most frequently as a means of protecting the basic needs and rights of people with mental disorders. Maintaining an exceptional, dedicated public mental health system ensures the existence of caregivers of last resort. Exceptionalism inspires the creation of special provisions—exceptions—in mainstream social insurance programs to protect people with mental disorders.[1] The most obvious example of such exceptionalism in mainstream social programs is the use of managed behavioral health care carve-out programs for Medicaid managed care arrangements.

Mainstreaming, by contrast, is advocated as a means of expanding the level and extent of mental health services and support for people with mental disorders. Our review of the past fifty years provides considerable evidence that is consistent with this argument. Inclusiveness and mainstreaming of people with even the most serious mental illnesses has resulted in tremendous gains in economic support for mental health care through SSI, SSDI, Medicare, and Medicaid.

The economic tide created by mainstreaming improved the economic circumstances of people with mental illness, but it swept the institutional structure of exceptionalism away with it. Most notably, the economic incentives set up by the Medicaid program motivated state mental health agencies (SMHAs) to surrender much of their policy authority, so as to increase the total funds available to support people with mental disorders. To maximize Medicaid revenue, SMHAs shifted elderly residents of public mental hospitals to nursing homes and gave priority to Medicaid-reimbursable services and Medicaid-eligible populations. The result today is that policy making about public mental health has moved, sometimes inadvertently, toward the leadership of the Medicaid program, which in most states is separate from the SMHA.

Obtaining more funds for mental health care through mainstreaming requires fitting people with mental disorders and mental health treatment into eligibility and service categories recognized by mainstream insurance and social programs. Mainstreaming has meant that people with mental illness depend on social insurance policies that are frequently applied uniformly across all types of beneficiaries, with little recognition of or accommodation to the special features of mental disorders and their treatment. Similarly, expanding private insurance coverage for mental health care has meant persuading regulators and payers that mental illness is "just like all other illnesses" and that treatment of mental disorders parallels the care of medical disorders.

The recent rhetoric of parity for private insurance coverage of mental health care provides a good example of how mainstreaming works and what its flaws are. Parity legislation seeks to extend the relatively generous insurance coverage held by the majority of Americans to mental illness, rather than enhancing specialized programs for people with severe mental disorders. Yet by defining parity as the same coverage for care of mental and other medical illnesses, this policy explicitly overlooks the sets of services that are unique to the care of severe mental disorders, such as day treatment, psychosocial rehabilitation, and vocational services (Frank et al., 2001).

Similar neglect of needs specific to mental health care affects both health insurance and social programs. Neither Medicare nor most private insurance policies have adapted their designs to incorporate scientific advances in the treatment of mental disorders by, for example, covering the treatment elements of collaborative care for depression. The recent implementation of return-to-work initiatives within the Social Security Income Support programs and some state provisions of Welfare to Work associated with the TANF program represent other examples where mainstreaming may disadvantage people with mental disorders.

Compelling mentally ill people to enter the labor force may not result in either increased work effort or poverty reduction.

Beyond these specific instances of policy failure is the more general problem that entry into the mainstream of the U.S. welfare state is simply not sufficient to prevent key segments of the population with mental illness from continued neglect and deprivation. Living in the community has special challenges and hazards for people with severe mental disorders. Their disorders may be associated with disturbed and disturbing behavior that can result in incarceration and eviction from stable housing arrangements (Jencks, 1994). The combination of poverty, limited access to housing, and severe mental illness can lead to increased vulnerability to crime and abuse. People with severe mental disorders continue to be overrepresented among homeless populations, among the population of inmates in U.S. jails and prisons, and among victims of crime and abuse. The onset of a severe and persistent mental illness still usually means that the affected individual faces a life of poverty. Although restoration and recovery are goals for people with mental disorders, it remains a distinct minority of people with severe and persistent mental disorders who realize these ends. Despite great advances, the probability of people with SPMI achieving stable, long-term employment that pays more than a subsistence wage is minute. Clinical science has not yet advanced to the point where recovery and reentry into the employed middle class can be an expectation of the majority of people with the most severe mental illnesses.

Building on Mainstreaming

For all but those with serious and persistent mental illnesses, mainstreaming—with certain modifications—has been a boon. Growth of private and public health insurance coverage, expansions in the scope of that coverage, and the substitution of managed care techniques for financial limits on coverage have led to increased rates of service use among those with less severe forms of mental illness. The development of more user-friendly treatments for many disorders has made treatment more effective and more acceptable. The provisions of the Americans with Disability Act may help people with less impairing conditions that tend to respond well to treatment maintain employment and guarantee other rights will be respected.

Many of the remaining problems faced by people in this group, including difficulties in obtaining appropriate treatment, are shared by people with other chronic disorders. For this group, further progress is likely to come through increasing the likelihood that people with these conditions will obtain effective and appropriate treatment. Here again the mainstream is likely to be the best source of future benefit. As in other areas of medical care, people with mental illness will gain from efforts to improve the quality and outcomes of treatment across providers and health plans. Incorporating treatment for mental illness into the scope of indicators that are routinely evaluated by mainstream purchasers and plans and including mental illness in pay-for-performance schemes is likely the best way to systematically improve treatment quality and, eventually, the well-being of this population.

New Institutional Structures

The overarching deficiency of mainstreaming is that it abandons the public responsibility for mental health care and the well-being of people with severe mental illnesses to a fragmented array of public programs that are run out of a large number of distinct federal, state, and local government bureaucracies. This fragmentation is in itself unexceptional. Under the best of circumstances, social insurance programs in the United States present potential beneficiaries with a complex array of inconsistent rules (Parrott and Dean, 2002). For people with severe mental disorders, whose illnesses inherently put them at a particular disadvantage in negotiating the maze of social program requirements, the fragmented social insurance system has especially deleterious effects on well-being.

How the presence of mental illnesses of different types affects eligibility, program requirements (e.g., work effort), and duration of benefits is highly variable. Those programs with an exceptionally high representation of people with mental illness, such as Medicaid, sometimes recognize special circumstances associated with mental illnesses. Most do not.

The policy challenge is to encourage the integration of people with mental disorders into the mainstream of U.S. society and social programs, at the same time recognizing unique features of their circumstances that federal, state, local, and private social and medical insurance programs must take into account to effectively serve them. This goal requires a new model of stewardship for the mental health system.

Historically, public mental hospitals and SMHAs formed the core of the mental health care delivery and support system. These identifiable agencies and institutions were visible to mental health care consumers, their families, and their advocates. SMHAs could be and were held politically accountable for mental health care. They were conduits for the voices of people with mental disorders and those interested in their well-being. They were the foundation of a mental health care system based on exceptionalism. Yet the cost of that specialized focal point was a system that had little general political support and was chronically underfunded.

As these institutions have lost financial authority over the past three decades, the challenge of creating a new model of stewardship has been an enduring topic for policy proposals. Most proposals during the 1980s and 1990s recommended expanding the reach of public mental health agencies at either the state or the local level (Talbott and Sharfstein, 1986; Mechanic, 1989; Shore and Cohen, 1990). The idea was to assign to a single public agency responsibility for managing diverse funding streams, treatment, and other forms of support and care for severely mentally ill people who are aided by public health, social, and income support programs. Looking backward, however, we can see that the track record of initiatives that placed a public mental health agency in a centralized planning role has been poor. These initiatives invariably became less able to maintain funding growth because they required continuous special pleadings; they became rigid because the voices of specialty mental health providers and mental health advocates were the only ones heard in decisions about program design; and they became progressively narrower because the specialty mental health sector frequently is limited in its expertise about the delivery of other human services (e.g., housing).

We should not reject mainstreaming, even for seriously mentally ill populations. The institutional foundations for future progress for people with serious mental disorders are the same as those that proved successful in the past—large, broad-based social and health insurance programs as well as the mainstream biomedical research enterprise.[2] Medicaid, Medicare, and Social Security are generally popular. They address a wide set of expanding needs in U.S. society. Even Medicaid, long associated with politically vulnerable means-tested social programs, has managed to grow in significance and continues to enjoy considerable political support (Brown and Sparer, 2003). The National Institutes of Health and the pharmaceutical industry have produced a series of major advances in treatment of mental disorders. We need to build a new stewardship structure that is consistent with mainstreaming.

This institutional structure needs to have several distinctive characteristics. First, the financial center of gravity in care and support of people with mental illness has moved to the federal level. Medicare, the Food Stamp program, SSDI, and much housing policy are purely federal. Most large employer health benefit plans are regulated exclusively by the federal government. Medicaid, SSI, and welfare are partnerships between the federal government and the states, with the federal government often establishing overarching rules that govern the allocation of funds. State governments remain critically important in mental health service delivery, and, as President Bush's New Freedom Commission (2003) suggested, mental health needs within states require enhanced governance. In addition, however, effective stewardship will require an institutional presence in the federal government. It is in the federal bureaucracy that a stewardship function will have the greatest opportunity for policy influence.

Second, progress has come through mainstream programs. Thus, a new federal stewardship institution should not administer or finance specialized mental health programs. Rather, it should take the form of introducing the concerns of people with serious and persistent mental illness and some corresponding elements of exceptionalism into larger social and health insurance agencies. It should advocate for the interests of people with mental illness and coordinate services among programs and across systems.

Third, many of the gains of the past fifty years have come about through the concerted efforts of people with mental illness and their families and supporters. A new agency should provide a locus for lobbying and advocacy efforts. It should channel the ideas and concerns of people with mental illness to the appropriate programmatic bureaucracy.

Fourth, the new institution needs to have a position within the federal bureaucracy that will provide it with authority. This implies that it should report directly to the president, rather than be subsumed within one of the departments or agencies whose activities it should be critiquing and coordinating. It further implies that the agency have some budgetary control. Though it would be inappropriate for an institution without programmatic authority to develop its own budgets, the new institution should have the ability to question or even veto agency appropriations focused on mental health.

The federal government contains a variety of structures that serve similar purposes, coordinating policy across diverse federal agencies. Over the past fifty years, such coordinating agencies have proliferated. The National Security Agency, the Council of Economic Advisors, and the National Economic Council all represent organizations aimed at assisting in coordination of information and decision making. All are advisory to the president and obtain their influence from that role, but they do not have any budgetary authority and do not influence policy at the state or local level.

One existing government entity that might serve as a model for housing a new mental health stewardship function is the Office of National Drug Control Policy (ONDCP). The ONDCP is charged with coordinating the array of federal agencies that participate in drug control to ensure that the activities of those agencies are consistent with the national drug control strategy. The ONDCP was created by 1988 legislation outlining a national drug control policy. The ONDCP was given a number of duties and several specific powers. Its first duty was to develop a national drug control strategy. Its second was to develop a budget for implementing that strategy. Its third duty was to oversee and coordinate implementation of the strategy by federal agencies (US GAO, 1999). The key power given to ONDCP in the 1988 act is to review the budgets of agencies involved in drug control and then to certify that the budgets are adequate to implement the drug control strategy. If ONDCP does not certify a budget, it must recommend spending plans or activities that would make the budget request adequate. The 1988 act states that agencies must comply with ONDCP recommendations before submitting final budget requests. This gives the views of the ONDCP a great deal of influence over the relevant federal agencies. This feature would offer a mechanism for aligning mental health policy across major federal programs (e.g., those of the SSA, Medicare, Substance Abuse and Mental Health Services Administration, HUD, and the Department of Education). It could also be used to implement the federal polices that affect programs such as TANF and Medicaid. This approach could not directly affect state and local government activities. Nevertheless, the significance of Medicaid, SSI, and the Alcohol, Drug Abuse, and Mental Health block grant for state funding of mental health care is sufficiently large (well over 50% of state-influenced spending); the new office overseeing mental health policy would probably be able effectively to signal states about policy priorities and their alignment with those policies.

Moving beyond the Mainstream

A federal agency to oversee the range of programs and regulations that may affect people with mental illness would be a significant step forward. It would institutionalize a voice for mental illness within the federal bureaucracy and enable mainstream policies to be tailored to the needs of people with mental illness. But a federal agency alone will not lift people with mental illness from poverty or ensure that their basic human needs are met.

Adding another layer of bureaucracy rarely improves the functioning of government. In this case, however, the proposed bureaucracy creates a locus of interest and responsibility at the federal level, where none now exists. Though the new agency may have limited capacity to take action, it should help in reorienting advocacy and interest group activity away from the states, whose powers are receding in this arena, and toward the federal government. Moreover, it should for the first time insert into the existing federal bureaucracy a voice for mental health.

People with serious and persistent mental illness can and do benefit from mainstream programs. Yet it is entirely feasible for society to do better still by this severely disadvantaged population.

Mainstream social welfare programs are always faced with a difficult trade-off. Increasing the generosity of benefits clearly improves the welfare of the beneficiary population. At the same time, more generous benefits attract people to social welfare programs. For example, increases in the generosity of SSDI benefits have led to a near tripling (an increase of 280%) of the beneficiary population over the past forty years (US SSA, 2004). Similarly, increases in the generosity of benefits discourage people receiving benefits from leaving social welfare programs when they are able to do so.

The very nature of serious and persistent mental illness makes these trade-offs easier to address in this group. The population with serious, persistent, and intractable mental illness is very small. People with these conditions are likely to have significant impairments in functioning, some beginning in early adulthood and lasting throughout their lives. Despite the advances of science over the past half century, most cannot be routinely and effectively cured of their symptoms and functional impairments. Although their functioning often cannot be fully restored, they benefit considerably from certain specialized services—such as supported housing, supported employment, and assertive community treatment. These services hold little appeal to people outside this group.

This pattern suggests that enhancement of services that benefit exclusively the population with mental illness—particularly supported housing—can achieve the twin aims of social welfare policy in this area. Increasing the availability of such housing will generate material improvements in the lives of people with mental illness. At the same time, few people in this group are likely to improve enough to be able to achieve a similar standard of living without recourse to this benefit, and the availability of supportive housing is not likely to lead to a large influx of nondisabled people seeking out this specialized social welfare benefit. By contrast, an increase in cash assistance, such as SSI benefits, would achieve the first goal but fail to achieve the second. An improvement in reimbursement for mental illness treatment might achieve the second and fail at the first.

Ideally, science will progress so that it is no longer necessary or appropriate to target programs to people with mental illness. In the interim, however, such enhanced benefits can substantially improve the welfare of people with mental illness at very little cost to society at large.

Conclusions

President Kennedy's mission was right, but his vision about how this might come about was wrong. We had to do better for people with mental illness, but the way we achieved that was primarily through the expansion of general social welfare programs and mainstream health insurance programs. These programs, together with improvements in treatment technologies, have made the lives of people with mental illness much better. But we must do better still.

The process of mainstreaming mental illness has eroded the institutional capacity to address the specific needs of this population. New institutional structures are needed to replace those that have disappeared. These institutional structures belong in the federal government, which is now the locus of control of most of the funds flowing to people with mental illness.

People with mental illness have benefited from mainstream programs in the past. They are likely to continue to benefit from these programs as the programs evolve in the future. Like other disabled populations, those with mental illness will benefit as disability insurance programs make it easier for people to collect benefits while reentering the labor market. Like other populations who have medical conditions, people with mental illness will benefit as mainstream health insurance programs become more adept at assessing and rewarding the quality of care delivered. Like other disadvantaged populations, people with mental illness will benefit as assistance levels increase.

The particularly disabling nature of severe and persistent mental illness means that we can—and should—do even better. By expanding social welfare programs that *exclusively* benefit a population that is permanently disabled, we can enhance their material well-being at little general cost. Given the extraordinary disability burden of the most severe mental illnesses, such steps are well worth taking.

Chapter Two • The Population with Mental Illness

1. For example, the incidence of breast cancer increased 4 percent per year between 1980 and 1987. Because this was a period of rapid adoption of mammography, the expanding use of new diagnostic technology—rather than changes in underlying health—is considered largely responsible for the dramatic rise in incidence (Garfinkel, Boring, and Heath, 1994).

2. These patterns are true of other conditions as well—many people with medical conditions do not get treatment for their conditions, and many people who seek treatment do not meet the criteria for specific medical conditions.

3. Even these refined estimates are probably flawed in that they are limited by the type of information available in surveys. For example, the effort to adjust the NCS survey estimates incorporated information not only on distress and functioning but also on use of services (Wakefield and Spitzer, 2002). The inclusion of information about use of services makes it difficult to use these refined estimates to assess unmet need for treatment.

4. Each demographic factor is best described as a correlate, not a cause, of a mental illness. Gender, for example, correlates with certain disorders (more women have depression, for example), but *gender* itself is not the cause. When any demographic factor correlates with an illness, it is usually difficult to infer the direction of causality from the observed correlations.

5. One difficulty in assessing the relationship between race and mental illness is the confounding effect of socioeconomic status. The lower socioeconomic status (SES) of blacks and other minorities might be a greater determinant of mental illness than their race. One early study found, for example, that within both the black and white populations, mental illness increases with decreasing SES (Hollingshead and Redlich, 1958). Today the prevailing view is that the prevalence of mental illness is similar across minority groups; any differences are more likely the result of SES or other factors (US DHHS CMHS, 1999, 2001a).

6. Though education level is not entirely free of this concern—mental illness frequently appears in the late teens and early twenties—it is likely less altered by mental illness than is an individual's income.

7. Dr. Leonard Scheele, then surgeon general of the United States, estimated in 1955 that 725,000 mentally ill patients were hospitalized for their conditions (*New York Times*, 1955). At the end of 1955 there were 560,000 resident patients in U.S. state and county mental hospitals, according to Grob (1991a, 260).

8. Again, the changes are similar to those for other diseases—the cutoff points for the diagnosis of high cholesterol have changed over time, as have the guidelines for the recommended daily allowance of various nutrients.

9. In 1973, for example, homosexuality was removed as a diagnosable disorder. (Ego-dystonic homosexuality continues to be listed, a disorder characterized by a pathological response to homosexual identity.) Other behaviors have been added to the list. For instance, with the 1979 publication of DSM-III, social phobia was described for the first time as a discernible type of phobia. Also introduced were somatization disorder (perhaps previously called hysteria or Briquet's syndrome), post-traumatic stress disorder (supplementing traumatic neuroses), and tobacco dependence.

10. The rate is even lower, 0.04 percent (defined as all psychoses, noninstitutionalized population only), in the 1957 Baltimore study.

11. A similar strategy has been used to project the future need for hospital beds (Goldsmith et al., 1993) and psychiatrists (Koran, 1979; Liptzin, 1979; Pardes, 1979). Kramer (1978, 1983) used similar methods to project the changing prevalence of schizophrenia and severe mental illness in the context of the changing sociodemographic composition of the U.S. population.

12. To the extent possible, we included only factors that are likely to cause (rather than follow) mental illness. We therefore excluded income and instead use individual education as a measure of socioeconomic status. To capture the idea that relative, rather than absolute, education is correlated with mental illness, we measured education in each census year relative to the mean in that year. Other variables included in the regression are gender, minority status, educational attainment, household composition, urbanness, and interactions between age and gender, age and race, race and gender, and race and education. Variables (main effects and interactions) were included if they were statistically significant predictors of symptoms or impairment.

Chapter Three • *The Evolving Technology of Mental Health Care*

1. The technological frontier reflects the best the system has to offer, rather than what is actually practiced or how faithfully it is practiced.

2. Comparative clinical trials offer the best, most direct comparisons of treatments from different eras. Yet because FDA approval requires that clinical trials show only efficacy against placebo rather than against earlier medications, comparative trials are not always performed. Clinical or comparative trials are even less frequent for new psychotherapies, partly because there is no FDA analogue to regulate their introduction. The dating of psychotherapy introduction is likely to be considerably less accurate than the dating of medication introduction because there is no regulatory mechanism like FDA approval.

3. *Exnovation* is a term used to describe the rejection of a previously adopted innovation (Rogers, 1995).

4. Since then, twelve clinical trials of such patients compared responses to clozapine versus older antipsychotics. A meta-analysis of those trials confirmed clozapine's superior overall efficacy, rate of compliance, and tolerability in terms of reducing EPS (Chakos et al., 2001).

5. For the subset of treatment-resistant patients, an efficacy advance has occurred with the newer antipsychotics.

6. "Obsessive compulsive reaction" was the nomenclature introduced by the first edition of the *Diagnostic and Statistical Manual,* or DSM-I (APA, 1952).

7. Dextroamphetamine, amphetamine, and methamphetamine.

8. Bipolar disorder also features a practice advance compared with the earlier era. Lithium remains the frontline treatment for bipolar disorder (APA, 2002). Lithium was not formally approved by FDA until 1970, but it was used in Europe in the 1950s and 1960s. One of psychiatry's first double-blind, placebo-controlled trials confirmed the Australian John Cade's finding of lithium as efficacious for symptomatic relief of mania (Schou, 1954). Further, the 1966 volume of the *American Handbook of Psychiatry* recognized the benefits of lithium and offered prescribing information in range with today's practice guidelines (Arieti, 1966). Anticonvulsants (e.g., valproate, lamotrigine) are now more widely used as frontline treatments, but they are a practice advance over lithium. Comparative clinical trials conducted in the 1990s established comparable efficacy between lithium and anticonvulsants, which are easier to prescribe and to tolerate (Blanco et al., 2002).

Chapter Four • Health Care Financing and Income Support

1. It should be noted that the availability of meaningful choice of ambulatory care for people with severe mental illnesses is complicated and frequently quite limited.

2. For recent data on this issue, see McAlpine and Mechanic (2000) and Sturm and Wells (2000).

3. *Social insurance* refers to income-replacement programs such as SSI and SSDI of the Social Security Administration.

4. Changes in the price of mental health care have always been important. Gerald Grob (1983) demonstrated how policy shifts between state and local governments first inhibited the growth and then promoted the expansion of public mental hospitals during the nineteenth century. From 1830 to 1890 state governments provided capital funds for the construction of public mental hospitals. Local governments were responsible for paying the variable costs of treating patients from their area. Thus, the price to local governments for state mental hospital services approximated the actual cost of each patient's care (i.e., the incremental cost of care). The price of care was high enough to discourage local governments from sending all but a small number of patients to state mental hospitals, whose census remained relatively low during the nineteenth century (Grob, 2001). Instead, local governments paid for care at local almshouses, which were cheaper but offered little active treatment.

The absence of active treatment in almshouses, and the growing demand to care for the most severely ill, prompted several states to pass legislation giving them sole responsibility for funding and providing care in state mental hospitals. New York and Massachusetts were the first states to assume full responsibility for care under the belief that local care not only was substandard, but also perpetuated chronicity and dependency. The shift to state-financed care dramatically reduced the price of mental health treatment to local governments. For them the price of state mental hospital care plummeted from the "true" incremental costs to zero.

The response to these legislative changes was enormous. From 1880 to 1920 the rate of admissions to local almshouses fell by 41 percent. The subset of elderly admissions over this period fell even more—by 77 percent. This was the first historical instance of trans-institutionalization of people with mental disorders. It also foretold the important role prices would play in the future in determining the setting and nature of mental health care in the United States.

5. The constraint on low-end matching serves to make the program less progressive and offers high-income states a relatively more attractive rate than what would be implied by a simple application of the matching rate formula.

6. Note that initially elderly persons were also excluded from Medicaid coverage in psychiatric hospitals, although this was later changed.

7. These figures were assembled from Reed (1975), Bureau of Labor Statistics Survey of Employee Health Benefits (various years), and A. Foster Higgins, Survey of Private Health Insurance Coverage (various years).

8. People with work-related disabilities may also receive workers' compensation payments.

9. Or, for those who become disabled before age thirty-one, an age-adjusted formula was used that required that they had worked at least six calendar quarters.

10. All events except insurance mandates were measured as dummy variables taking on a value of one from the effective date of the policy and after. Mandates were measured as a cumulative count of the states that enacted mandated minimum benefit statutes (eventually including parity laws).

Chapter Five • *The Supply of Mental Health Services*

1. We are grateful to Saul Feldman for his personal reflections on the development of this industry. See his *Managed Behavioral Health Services* (2003).

2. To obtain occupancy rate estimates, we used the ratio of resident patients at the end of the year divided by the reported number of beds in private psychiatric hospitals. All data were taken from chapter 14 of *Mental Health, United States, 2000 (US DHHS, CMHS, 2001b)*.

Chapter Six • *Policy Making in Mental Health*

1. The statement in 1961 by the JCMIH offered a conclusion that has become a modern refrain: the therapeutic possibilities in mental health are far better than the outcomes actually realized. The failure of the mental health system to achieve its potential stems from barriers to accessing treatment and the inappropriate care of many who enter treatment (JCMIH, 1961; US DHHS, CMHS, 1999).

2. The CMHC grant mechanism was modified to pay for operating expenses for a limited time and for training of mental health workers.

3. See, for example, www.usdoj.gov/crt/split/documents/cshsa.htm.

4. See the Department of Health and Human Services Web sites, including SAMHSA. gov, ssa.gov, and cms.gov.

5. This is due partly to the design of the case-management function but it is also due to the limits on effective choice of providers for people with Medicaid when outpatient fees are set below private market levels (see Frank and Goldman, 1989, for a detailed discussion of these issues).

6. Among this group of policy entrepreneurs were Pam Hyde, Martha Knisely, Michael Hogan, Dennis Jones, and Steven Mayburg.

Chapter Seven • *Assessing the Well-being of People with Mental Illness*

1. To confirm that the observed patterns did not arise as a consequence of changes in the underlying prevalence of mental illness, we also plotted diagnosis patterns for specific cohorts: adults born between 1945 and 1954 and children born between 1968 and 1973. In both cases, the patterns were the same within cohorts as for the population as a whole. Finally, we examined data for the nonwhite population. Again, the pattern was quite similar to that plotted in the figures.

2. The data show a modest increase in the percentage of patients with psychiatric symptoms who were given a psychiatric diagnosis (from about 57% in 1977 to about 68% in the late 1990s). This increase is offset, however, by an increase in the share of patients who reported psychiatric symptoms (from about 3.5% in the late 1970s to about 4.5% in the late 1980s), so the percentage of patients with psychiatric symptoms who did not receive a diagnosis has remained steady over time.

3. One concern about changes in prevalence of treatment rates is that increases may reflect errors of diagnosis, rather than better case identification. Some evidence suggests that the quality of psychiatric diagnosis in medical care has been improving rather than declining over time. Our analysis of the NAMCS shows increases in the propensity to diagnose mental illness among most PCPs, and not only among a few who treat substantial numbers of patients with mental disorders. Furthermore, physicians are increasingly likely to diagnose mental illness in patients presenting with mental health symptoms. Conversely, the rate at which physicians ascribe mental health diagnoses to patients with somatic illnesses only has been declining.

4. This increase is mainly a consequence of an increase in the out-of-pocket share of hospital costs. The difference in spending patterns between 1987 and 1996 may also reflect a difference in the severity of cases, which is consistent with the increase in the prevalence of diagnosed mental illness documented from 1987 (NMES) to 1996 (MEPS). To address this possibility, we compared the mental health expenditures of the most severely ill individuals in each sample, those with schizophrenia or other psychotic conditions. Because these are the most serious conditions, the individuals probably represent cases of similar severity. Total health expenditures for severely ill persons were $4,006 (1996 dollars) in 1987; of that amount $2,397 was spent on mental health care, 18 percent of which was paid

out of pocket. In the 1996 sample total health expenditures were $8,941 for this group, $7,124 having been spent on mental health care, 8 percent of which was paid out of pocket. These analyses are based on very small samples, but they do support our general findings of increased financial protection.

5. In 1970 Linn et al. (1977) documented that a sample of patients who moved from hospital to community-based living arrangements were more satisfied with their overall life conditions than were those who stayed in the hospital. In the early 1980s Lehman et al. (1982) found that patients reported higher levels of satisfaction with board and care homes than with hospitalization, principally because those settings gave them privacy and greater contact with their families. In an examination comparing patients in the hospital to those in the community, Lehman et al. (1986) found that community residents viewed their living conditions more favorably, had more financial resources, and were less likely to suffer from personal injury from assault. Studies from the 1990s confirm and supplement these earlier results. Rosenfield (1992) showed that conditions that increase the level of control perceived by people with SPMI increase their subjective quality of life. Schutt et al. (1997) and Marshall et al. (1996) found that homeless people with mental illness were more satisfied with their living conditions after moving into permanent residences and preferred independent housing to group living arrangements.

6. Stigma is manifested as bias, distrust, stereotyping, fear, embarrassment, anger, or avoidance—or a combination of these (*US DHHS, CMHS,* 1999). Persons with mental illnesses seek to avoid stigma and rejection by concealing their disorders. In addition, stigma affects the self-esteem of those with mental illnesses, creates barriers to seeking care, and affects the course of treatment (Wahl, 1999; Sirey et al., 2001). Further, stigma may result in restrictions on the civil liberties of persons with mental illness and limits on insurance coverage for mental health services (Hanson, 1998; Pescosolido et al., 1999; McSween, 2002).

7. For instance, rather than asking about mental illnesses, many surveys conducted in the 1950s and 1960s referred to nervous breakdowns.

8. We made limited use of other older surveys with measures that were similar to more recent surveys and pointed to cases in which different wording made comparisons difficult.

9. For our purposes, we set aside the issue that media coverage may be a *cause* of stigma and instead used media content as an *indicator* of popular perceptions.

10. The 1996 GSS repeated an open-ended question from an earlier study that used a similar methodology and sampling frame (Star, 1952, 1955).

Chapter Eight • Looking Forward

1. See, for examples, the recent discussion of the Social Security Administration's Ticket to Work program (Salkever, 2003).

2. Interestingly, leaders in psychiatric research made a similar calculation in separating NIMH's service and research functions and returning the NIMH and its research to the National Institutes of Health.

American Academy of Pediatrics. 2001. Clinical practice guideline: Treatment of the school aged child with attention deficit-hyperactivity disorder. *Pediatrics* 108(4):1033–44.

American Medical Association. 1978, 1980, 1981. *Profile of Medical Practice*. Chicago: American Medical Association.

———. 1987–93. *Directory of Graduate Medical Education Programs*. Chicago: American Medical Association.

———. 1981–84, 1986–87, 1990, 1992, 1995–2000. *Physician Characteristics and Distribution in the U.S.* Chicago: American Medical Association.

———. 1983–97. *Socioeconomic Characteristics of Medical Practice*. Chicago: American Medical Association.

———. 1995, 1996, 1997–98. *Physician Marketplace Statistics: Profiles for Detailed Specialties, Selected States and Practice Arrangements*. Chicago: American Medical Association, Center for Health Policy Research.

———. 1999. *Physician Socioeconomic Statistics*. Chicago: American Medical Association, Center for Health Policy Research.

American Psychiatric Association. 1952. *Diagnostic and Statistical Manual of Mental Disorders*. 1st ed. (DSM-I). Washington, D.C.: American Psychiatric Association.

———. 1968. *Diagnostic and Statistical Manual of Mental Disorders*. 2nd ed. (DSM-II). Washington, D.C.: American Psychiatric Association.

———. 1979. *Diagnostic and Statistical Manual of Mental Disorders*. 3rd ed. (DSM-III). Washington, D.C.: American Psychiatric Association.

———. 1987. *Diagnostic and Statistical Manual of Mental Disorders*. 3rd ed., rev. (DSM-III-R). Washington, D.C.: American Psychiatric Association.

———. 1993. Practice guideline for major depressive disorder in adults. *American Journal of Psychiatry* 150 (Suppl. 4):1–26.

———. 1994a. *Diagnostic and Statistical Manual of Mental Disorders*. 4th ed. (DSM-IV). Washington, D.C.: American Psychiatric Association.

———. 1994b. Practice guidelines for the treatment of patients with bipolar disorder. *American Journal of Psychiatry* 151 (12 Suppl.):1–36.

———. 1998. Practice guidelines for the treatment of patients with panic disorder. *American Journal of Psychiatry* 155(5):1–34.

———. 2000. *Diagnostic and Statistical Manual of Mental Disorders*. 4th ed., rev. (DSM-IV-TR). Washington, D.C.: American Psychiatric Association.

———. 2002. Practice guidelines for the treatment of patients with bipolar disorder (rev.). *American Journal of Psychiatry* 159 (4 Suppl.):1–50.

Anderson, I. M., and B. M. Tomenson. 1995. Treatment discontinuation with selective serotonin reuptake inhibitors compared with tricyclic anti-depressants: A meta-analysis. *BMJ* 10:1433–38.

Angermeyer, M. C., and H. Matschinger. 1996. The effect of violent attacks by schizophrenic persons on the attitude of the public towards the mentally ill. *Social Science and Medicine* 43(12):1721–28.

Angst, J. 1961. A clinical analysis of the effects of Tofranil in depression: Longitudinal and follow-up studies. Treatment of blood-relations. *Psychopharmacologia* 2:381–40.

Arieti, S., ed. 1959. *American Handbook of Psychiatry*, vols. 1–2. New York: Basic Books.

———. 1966. *American Handbook of Psychiatry*, vol. 3. New York: Basic Books.

Arrow, K. J. 1963. Uncertainty and the welfare economics of medical care. *American Economic Review* 53(5):941–73.

Ashbaugh, J. W., P. J. Leaf,. R. W. Manderscheid, and W. Eaton. 1983. Estimates of the size and selected characteristics of the adult chronically mentally ill population living in US households. *Research in Community and Mental Health* 3:3–24.

Ashbaugh, J. W., and R. W. Manderscheid. 1985. A method for estimating the chronic mentally ill population in state and local areas. *Hospital and Community Psychiatry* 36(4):389–93.

Autor, D. H., and M. G. Duggan. 2003. The rise in disability rolls and the decline in unemployment. *Quarterly Journal of Economics* 118(1):157–205.

Baldessarini, R., and F. R. Frankenburg. 1991. Clozapine: A novel antipsychotic agent. *New England Journal of Medicine* 324:746–54.

Ballenger, J. C., G. D. Burrows, R. L. DuPont, et al. 1998. Alprazolam and panic disorder and agoraphobia: Results from a multicenter trial. I. Efficacy in short-term treatment. *Archives of General Psychiatry* 45(5):413–22.

Ballenger, J. C., J. R. Davidson, Y. Lecrubier, et al. 1998. Consensus statement on social anxiety disorder from the International Consensus Group on Depression and Anxiety. *Journal of Clinical Psychiatry* 59 (Suppl. 17):54–60.

Ballenger, J. C., and R. M. Post. 1978. Therapeutic effects of carbamazepine in affective illness: A preliminary report. *Community Psychopharmacology* 2:159–75.

Barker, P. R., R. W. Manderscheid, and G. E. Hendershot. 1992. Serious mental illness and disability in the adult household population: United States, 1989. In U.S. Department of Health and Human Services, Center for Mental Health Services, *Mental Health, United States, 1992*, ed. R. W. Manderscheid and M. A. Sonnenschein. Rockville, Md.: Substance Abuse and Mental Health Services Administration, Center for Mental Health Services, 255–88.

Barlow, D. H., M. G. Craske, J. A. Cerny, and J. S. Klosko. 1989. Behavioral treatment of panic disorder. *Behavior Therapy* 20:261–82.

Bartel, A., and P. Taubman. 1979. Health and labor market success: The role of various diseases. *Review of Economics and Statistics* 61(1):1–8.

———. 1986. Some economic and demographic consequences of mental illness. *Journal of Labor Economics* 4(2):243–56.

Bazelon Center for Mental Health Law. 2002. *Civil Rights and Human Dignity: Three Decades of Leadership in Advocacy for People with Mental Disabilities.* Washington, D.C.: Judge David L. Bazelon Center for Mental Health Law.

Beck, A. 1976. *Cognitive Therapy and the Emotional Disorders.* New York: Meridian Press.

Berk, M., L. Ichim, and S. Brook. 1999. Olanzapine compared to lithium in mania: A double-blind randomized controlled trial. *International Clinical Psychopharmacology* 14:339–43.

Berndt, E. R., A. Bir, S. H. Busch, et al. 2002. The medical treatment of depression, 1991–1996: Productive inefficiency, expected outcome variations, and price indexes. *Journal of Health Economics* 21(3):373–96.

Berndt, E. R., S. H. Busch, and R. G. Frank. 2000/2001. Interpreting changes in mental health expenditures: Minding our Ps and Qs. *NBER Reporter,* Winter.

Bird, H. R., T. J. Yager, B. Staghezza, et al. 1990. Impairment in the epidemiological measurement of psychopathology in the community. *Journal of the American Academy of Child and Adolescent Psychiatry* 29:796–803.

Blanco, C., G. Laje, M. Olfson, et al. 2002. Trends in the treatment of bipolar disorder by outpatient psychiatrists. *American Journal of Psychiatry* 159(6):1005–10.

Borinstein, A. B. 1992. Public attitudes toward persons with mental illness. *Health Affairs* 11(3):186–96.

Bowden, C. L., A. M. Brugger, A. C. Swann, et al. 1994. Efficacy of Divalproex versus lithium and placebo in the treatment of mania. *Journal of the American Medical Association* 271:918–24.

Bradley, C. 1937. The behavior of children receiving benzedrine. *American Journal of Psychiatry* 94:577–85.

Bradley, C., and M. Bowen. 1940. School performance of children receiving amphetamine (benzedrine) sulfate. *American Journal of Orthopsychiatry* 10:782–89.

Brown, L. D., and M. S. Sparer. 2003. Poor program's progress: The unanticipated politics of Medicaid policy. *Health Affairs* 22(1):31–44.

Bruzzese, A. 1989. Double-digit increase per worker hits health costs. *Employee Benefit News,* March.

Bureau of Labor and Statistics, National Compensation Survey. *Employee Benefits in Private Industry in the United States.* Bulletin 2140 (1982), Bulletin 2176 (1983), Bulletin 2281 (1987), Bulletin 2236 (1989), and 2002 report. Washington, D.C.: Bureau of Labor Statistics.

Burt, M. R. 1992. *Over the Edge: The Growth of Homelessness in the 1980s.* Washington, D.C.: Urban Institute Press.

———. 2001. What will it take to end homelessness? *Urban Institute Brief,* October.

Busch, S. H., E. R. Berndt, and R. G. Frank. 2001. Creating price indexes for measuring productivity in mental health care. In *Frontiers of Health Policy,* vol. 4, ed. A. Garber. Chicago: University of Chicago Press for the National Bureau of Economic Research.

Cade, J. 1949. Lithium salts in the treatment of psychotic excitement. *Medical Journal of Australia* 2:349–52.

Carlsson, A., H. Corrodi, K. Fuxe, and T. Hokfelt. 1969. Effect of antidepressant drugs on the depletion of intraneuronal brain 5-hydroxytryptamine stores caused by 4-methyl-alpha-ethyl-meta-tyramine. *European Journal of Pharmacology* 5(4):357–66.

Casey, J., I. Bennett, C. J. Lindley, et al. 1960. Drug therapy in schizophrenia. A controlled study of the relative effectiveness of chlorpromazine, promazine, phenobarbital, and placebo. *Archives of General Psychiatry* 2:210–20.

Casey, J., J. Lasky, C. Klett, and L. Hollister. 1960. Treatment of schizophrenic reactions with phenothiazine derivatives: A comparative study of chlorpromazine, triflupromazine, mepazine, prochlorperazine, perphenazine, and phenobarbital. *American Journal of Psychiatry* 117:97–105.

Chakos, M., J. Lieberman, E. Hoffman, et al. 2001. Effectiveness of second-generation antipsychotics in patients with treatment-resistant schizophrenia: A review and meta-analysis of randomized trial. *American Journal of Psychiatry* 158:518–26.

Chang, C. F., L. J. Kiser, J. E. Bailey, et al. 1998. Tennessee's failed managed care program for mental health and substance abuse services. *Journal of the American Medical Association* 279(11):864–69.

Clark, D. M., P. M. Salkovskis, A. Hackmann, et al. 1994. A comparison of cognitive therapy, applied relaxation and imipramine in the treatment of panic disorder. *British Journal of Psychiatry* 164(6):759–69.

Clark, R. F., J. Turek-Brezina, C. Hawes, and C. Chu. 1994. *Licensed Board and Care Home: Preliminary Findings from the 1991 National Health Provider Inventory.* Washington, D.C.: U.S. Department of Health and Human Services.

Clausen, J. A. 1956. *Sociology and the Field of Mental Health.* New York: Russell Sage Foundation.

Coffey, R. M., T. Mark, E. King, et al. 2000. *National Expenditures for Mental Health and Substance Abuse Treatment, 1997.* SAMHSA Publication SMA-00-3499. Rockville, Md.: Substance Abuse and Mental Health Services Administration.

Cole, N. J., C. H. H. Branch, and M. Orla. 1957. Mental illness. *Archives of Neurology and Psychiatry* 77:393–98.

Commission on Chronic Illness. 1957. *Chronic Illness in the United States.* Cambridge: Harvard University Press.

Costello, E. J., A. Angold, B. J. Burns, et al. 1996. The Great Smoky Mountains Study of Youth: Goals, design, methods, and the prevalence of DSM-III-R disorders. *Archives of General Psychiatry* 53(12): 1129–36.

Council of Economic Advisers. 2002. *Economic Report of the President.* Washington, D.C.: U.S. Government Printing Office.

Council on Social Work Education. 1977. *Statistics on Social Work Education in the United States.* Alexandria, Va.: Council on Social Work Education.

———. 1998. *Statistics on Social Work Education in the United States.* Alexandria, Va.: Council on Social Work Education.

Coverdale, J., R. Nairn, and D. Claasen. 2002. Depictions of mental illness in print media: A prospective national sample. *Australian and New Zealand Journal of Psychiatry* 36:697–700.

Cronkite, K. 1995. *On the Edge of Darkness: Conversations about Conquering Depression.* New York: Dell.

Cross-National Collaborative Group. 1992. The changing rate of major depression: Cross-national comparisons. *Journal of the American Medical Association* 268(21):3098–105.

Deutsch, Albert. *The Shame of the States.* New York: Harcourt, Brace, 1948.

Diamond, P. M., E. W. Wang, C. E. Holzer III, et al. 2001. The prevalence of mental illness in prison. *Administration and Policy in Mental Health and Mental Health Services Research* 29(1):21–40.

Dickey, B., P. R. Binner, S. Leff, et al. 1989. Containing mental health treatment costs through program design: A Massachusetts study. *American Journal of Public Health* 79(7):863–67.

DiMasi, J. A., and L. Lasagna. 1995. The economics of psychotropic drug development. In *Psychopharmacology: 4th Generation of Progress.* American College of Neuropsychopharmacology. New York: Raven Press, 1883–95.

Dohrenwend, B. P., and E. Chin-Shong. 1967. Social status and attitudes toward psychological disorder: The problem of tolerance and deviance. *American Sociological Review* 32(3):417–33.

Dohrenwend, B. P., G. Egri, and F. S. Mendelsohn. 1971. Psychiatric disorder in general populations: A study of the problem of clinical judgment. *American Journal of Psychiatry* 127:1304–12.

Dolnick, E. 1998. *Madness on the Couch: Blaming the Victim in the Heyday of Psychoanalysis.* New York: Simon and Schuster.

Donelly, G. 1980.Psychosurgery. In *Comprehensive Textbook of Psychiatry,* 3rd ed., ed. H. I. Kaplan, A. M. Freedman, and B. J. Sadock. Baltimore: Williams and Wilkins, 2342–48.

Dulcan, M., and the Work Group on Quality Issues. 1997. Practice parameters for the assessment and treatment of children, adolescents, and adults with attention-deficit/hyperactivity disorder. *Journal of the American Academy of Child and Adolescent Psychiatry* 36 (10 Suppl.):85S–121S.

Eaton, J. W., and R. J. Weil. 1955. *Culture and Mental Disorders.* Glencoe, Ill.: Free Press.

Eaton, W., J. Anthony, J. Gallo, et al. 1997. Natural history of diagnostic interview schedule/DSM-IV major depression: The Baltimore Epidemiologic Catchment Area follow-up. *Archives of General Psychiatry* 54(11):993–99.

Emrich, H. M., D. von Zerssen, and W. Kissling. 1981. On a possible role of gap in mania: therapeutic efficacy of sodium valproate. In *Data and Benzodiazepine Receptors,* ed. E. Costa, G. Dicharia, and G. L. Gessa. New York: Raven Press, 287–96.

Endicott, J., and R. L. Spitzer. 1978. A diagnostic interview: The Schedule for Affective Disorders and Schizophrenia. *American Journal of Psychiatry* 25:131–39.

Ettner, S. L., R. G. Frank, and R. C. Kessler. 1997. The impact of psychiatric disorder on labor market outcomes. *Industrial and Labor Relations Review* 51(1):64–81.

Ettner, S. L., and E. H. Notman. 1997. How well do ambulatory care groups predict expenditures of mental health and substance abuse patients? *Journal of Administration and Policy in Mental Health* 24(4):339–58.

Eysenck, H. 1952. The effects of psychotherapy: An evaluation. *Journal of Consulting Psychology* 16:319–24.

———. 1965. The effects of psychotherapy. *International Journal of Psychiatry* 1:99–144.

Fein, R. 1958. *Economics of Mental Illness.* New York: Basic Books.

Feldman, S. 2002. Choices and challenges. In *Managed Behavioral Health Services: Perspectives and Practices,* ed. S. Feldman. Springfield, Ill.: Charles C. Thomas, 3–23.

Felix, R. H. 1965. *Mental Illness: Progress and Prospects.* New York: Columbia University Press.

Ferguson, T. W. 1990. Any wonder medical premiums are anything but shrinking. *Wall Street Journal*, 22 May.

Foa, E. B., and M. J. Kozak. 1986. Emotional processing of fear: Exposure to corrective information. *Psychological Bulletin* 99:20–35.

Foa, E. B., G. Steketee, M. J. Kozak, and D. Dugger. 1987. Effects of imipramine on depression and obsessive-compulsive symptoms. *Psychiatry Research* 21:123–36.

Fombonne, E. 1994. Increased rates of depression: Update of epidemiological findings and analytical problems. *Acta Psychiatrica Scandinavica* 90:145–56.

Foote, S. M., and C. Hogan. 2001. Disability profile and health care costs of Medicare beneficiaries under age sixty-five. *Health Affairs* 20(6):242–53.

Foster, P. S., and R. M. Eisler. 2001. An integrated approach to the treatment of obsessive-compulsive disorder. *Comprehensive Psychiatry* 42:24–31.

Foster Higgins National Survey of Employer Sponsored Health Plans. 1995, 1997, 1999. Washington, D.C.: A. Foster Higgins and Co.

Frank, J. 1961. *Persuasion and Healing: A Comparative Study of Psychotherapy.* Baltimore: Johns Hopkins University Press.

Frank, R. G. 1985. A model of state expenditures on mental hospital services. *Public Finance Quarterly* 13(3):319–38.

———. 1989a. Regulatory policy and information deficiencies in the market for mental health services. *Journal of Health Politics, Policy and Law* 14(3):477–503.

———. 1989b. Regulatory responses to information deficiencies in the market for mental health services. In *The Future of Mental Health Services Research*, ed. C. A. Taube, D. Mechanic, and A. A. Hohmann. Rockville, Md.: U.S. Department of Health and Human Services, 113–38.

———. 2000. The creation of Medicare and Medicaid: The emergence of insurance and markets for mental health services. *Psychiatric Services* 51(4):465–68.

Frank, R. G., E. R. Berndt, A. B. Busch, and A. F. Lehman. 2004. Price indexes for the ongoing treatment of schizophrenia: An exploratory study. *Quarterly Review of Economics and Finance* 44(3):390–409.

Frank, R. G., and P. Gertler. 1991. An assessment of measurement error bias for estimating the impact of mental distress on earnings. *Journal of Human Resources* 26(1):154–64.

Frank, R. G., and H. H. Goldman. 1989. Financing care of the severely mentally ill: Incentives, contracts and public responsibility. *Journal of Social Issues* 45(3):131–44.

Frank, R. G., H. H. Goldman, and M. Hogan. 2003. Medicaid and mental health: Be careful what you ask for. *Health Affairs* 22(1):101–13.

Frank, R.G., H. H. Goldman, and T. G. McGuire. 2001. Will parity in coverage result in better mental health care? *New England Journal of Medicine* 345(23):1701–4.

Frank, R. G., and J. Lave. 2003. Economics. In *Managed Behavioral Health Services: Perspectives and Practices*, ed. S. Feldman. Springfield, Ill.: Charles C. Thomas, 101–26.

Frank, R. G., and T. G. McGuire. 2000. Economics and mental health. In *Handbook of Health Economics*, ed. J. P. Newhouse and A. Culyer. New York: Elsevier.

Frank, R. G., T. G. McGuire, and J. P. Newhouse. 1995. Risk contracts in managed mental health care. *Health Affairs* 14(3):50–64.

Frank, R. G., T. G. McGuire, S. L. Normand, and H. H. Goldman. 1999. The value of mental health services at the systems level: The case of treatment for depression. *Health Affairs* 18(5):71–88.

Frank, R. G., D. S. Salkever, and S. S. Sharfstein. 1991. A look at rising mental health insurance costs. *Health Affairs* 10(2):116–24.

Freedman, A. M., and H. I. Kaplan, eds. 1967. *Comprehensive Textbook of Psychiatry*. Baltimore: Williams and Wilkins.

Garfinkel, L., C. C. Boring, and C. W. Heath Jr. 1994. Changing trends. An overview of breast cancer incidence and mortality. *Cancer* 74 (1 Suppl.):222–27.

Geddes, J., N. Freemantle, P. Harrison, and P. Bebbington. 2000. Atypical antipsychotics in the treatment of schizophrenia: Systematic overview and meta-regression analysis. *BMJ* 321(7273):1371–76.

Gelernter, C. S., T. W. Uhde, P. Cimbolic, et al. 1991. Cognitive-behavioral and pharmacological treatments of social phobia: A controlled study. *Archives of General Psychiatry* 48(2):938–45.

Geller, J. L. 2000. The last half-century of psychiatric services as reflected in psychiatric services. *Psychiatric Services* 51(1):41–67.

Geoghegan, J. J., and G. H. Stevenson. 1949. Prophylactic electroshock. *American Journal of Psychiatry* 105:494.

Goldman, H. 1977. Conflict, competition, and coexistence: The mental hospital as parallel health and welfare systems. *American Journal of Orthopsychiatry* 47(1):60–65.

Goldman, H. H., N. H. Adams, and C. A. Taube. 1983. Deinstitutionalization: The data demythologized. *Hospital and Community Psychiatry* 34(2):129–34.

Goldman, H. H., and A. A. Gattozzi. 1988. *Murder in the Cathedral* revisited: President Reagan and the mentally disabled. *Hospital and Community Psychiatry* 39(3):505–9.

Goldman, H. H., S. Thelander, and C.-G. Westrin. 2000. Organizing mental health services: An evidence-based approach. *Journal of Mental Health Policy and Economics* 3:69–75.

Goldsmith, H. F., R. W. Manderscheid, M. J. Henderson, and A. J. Sacks. 1993. Projections of inpatient admissions to specialty mental health organizations, 1990–2010. *Hospital and Community Psychiatry* 44(5):478–83.

Grob, G. 1983. *Mental Illness and American Society, 1875–1940*. Princeton: Princeton University Press.

———. 1991a. *From Asylum to Community: Mental Health Policy in Modern America*. Princeton.: Princeton University Press

———. 1991b. Origins of DSM-I: A study in appearance and reality. *American Journal of Psychiatry* 148(4):421–31.

———. 1994. *The Mad among Us: A History of the Care of America's Mentally Ill*. Cambridge: Harvard University Press.

Grob, G. 2001. Mental health policy in twentieth-century America. In U.S. Department of Health and Human Services, Center for Mental Health Services, *Mental Health, United States, 2000*, ed. R. W. Manderscheid and M. J. Henderson. DHHS Publication (SMA) 01-3537. Rockville, Md.: Substance Abuse and Mental Health Services Administration, Center for Mental Health Services, 3–14.

Gronfein, W. 1985. Incentives and intentions in mental health policy: A comparison of the Medicaid and community mental health programs. *Journal of Health and Social Behavior* 26:192–206.

Hall, B., and B. Khan. 2003. Adoption of new technologies. In *New Economy Handbook*, ed. D. Jones. Amsterdam: Elsevier Science, chap. 10.

Hallowell, E., and J. J. Ratey. 1994. *Driven to Distraction*. New York: Pantheon.

Hanson, K. W. 1998. Public opinion and the mental health parity debate: Lessons from the survey literature. *Psychiatric Services* 49(8):1059–66.

Harkness, J. S., S. Newman, and D. Salkever. 2004. The cost effectiveness of independent housing for the chronically mentally ill: Do housing and neighbourhood features matter? *Health Services Research* 39(5):1141–60.

Hartigan, G. P. 1963. The use of lithium salts in affective disorders. *British Journal of Psychiatry* 190:810.

Hogan, L. L. 1981. *Subsidized Programs for Low-Income People*. New Brunswick, N.J.: Transaction Books.

Hogarty, G. E., and S. C. Goldberg. 1973. Drug and sociotherapy in aftercare schizophrenic patients. *Archives of General Psychiatry* 28:54–65.

Hollingshead, A. B., and F. C. Redlich. 1958. *Social Class and Mental Illness: A Community Study*. New York: Wiley.

Horvitz-Lennon, M., S. L. T. Normand, P. Gaccione, and R. G. Frank. 2001. Partial versus full hospitalization for adults in psychiatric distress: A systematic review of the published literature (1957–1997). *American Journal of Psychiatry* 158(5):676–85.

Huskamp, H. A., P. A. Deverka, A. M. Epstein, et al. 2003. The effect of incentive-based formularies on prescription-drug utilization and spending. *New England Journal of Medicine* 349(23):2224–32.

Hyde, R. W., and L. V. Kingsley. 1944. Studies in medical sociology: The relation of mental disorder to the community socioeconomic level. *New England Journal of Medicine* 231:543–48.

Jacobsen, K., T. G. McGuire, and E. H. Notman. 1996. Organizational structure and state mental health expenditures. *Administration and Policy in Mental Health* 23(6):475–92.

Jencks, C. 1994. *The Homeless*. Cambridge: Harvard University Press.

Jensen, P. S., S. P. Hinshaw, J. M. Swanson, et al. 2001. Findings from the NIMH Multimodal Treatment Study of ADHD (MTA): Implications and applications for primary care providers. *Journal of Developmental and Behavioral Pediatrics* 22(1):60–73.

Joint Commission on Mental Illness and Health. 1961. *Action for Mental Health: Final Report*. New York: Basic Books.

Kane, J. M., G. Honingfeld, J. Singer, H. Meltzer, and Clozaril Collaborative Study Group. 1988. Clozapine for the treatment-resistant schizophrenic: A double blind comparison with chlorpromazine. *Archives of General Psychiatry* 45:780–96.

Kaplan H. I., A. M. Freedman, and B. J. Sadock, eds. 1980. *Comprehensive Textbook of Psychiatry*. 3rd ed. Baltimore: Williams and Wilkins.

Kaplan, H. I., and B. J. Sadock, eds. 1985. *Comprehensive Textbook of Psychiatry*. 4th ed. Baltimore: Williams and Wilkins.

———. 1989. *Comprehensive Textbook of Psychiatry*. 5th ed. Baltimore: Williams and Wilkins.

———. 1995. *Comprehensive Textbook of Psychiatry*. 6th ed. Baltimore: Williams and Wilkins.

Katon, W. 1993. *Panic Disorder in the Medical Setting.* NIH Publication 93–3482. Rockville, Md.: National Institutes of Health.

Kelleher, K., M. Chaffin, J. Hollenberg, and E. Fischer. 1994. Alcohol and drug disorders among physically abusive and neglectful parents in a community-based sample. *American Journal of Public Health* 84:1586–90.

Keller, M. B., G. L. Klerman, P. W. Lavori, et al. 1982. Treatment received by depressed patients. *Journal of the American Medical Association* 248(15):1848–55.

Keller, M. B., P. W. Lavori, G. L. Klerman, et al. 1986. Low levels and lack of predictors of somatotherapy and psychotherapy received by depressed patients. *Archives of General Psychiatry* 43(5):458–66.

Kennedy, J. F. 1963. *Message from the President of the United States Relative to Mental Illness and Mental Retardation.* Washington, D.C.: U.S. Government Printing Office.

Kent, J. M., J. D. Coplan, and J. M. Gorman. 1998. Clinical utility of the selective serotonin reuptake inhibitors in the spectrum of anxiety. *Biological Psychiatry* 44:812–24.

Kessler, D. A., P. A. Berglund, M. L. Bruce, et al. 2001. The prevalence and correlates of untreated serious mental illness. *Health Services Research* 36(6):987–1007.

Kessler, D., and M. McClellan. 2002. Ownership form and trapped capital in the hospital industry. NBER working paper w8989. National Bureau of Economic Research.

Kessler, R. C., P. Berglund, E. E. Walters, et al. 1998. Population-based analyses: A methodology for estimating the twelve-month prevalence of serious mental illness. In U.S. Department of Health and Human Services, Center for Mental Health Services, *Mental Health, United States, 1998*, ed. R. W. Manderscheid and M. J. Henderson. Rockville, Md.: Substance Abuse and Mental Health Services Administration, Center for Mental Health Services, 99–109.

Kessler, R. C., W. T. Chiu, O. Demler, and E. E. Walters. 2005. Prevalence, severity, and comorbidity of 12-month DSM-IV disorders in the National Comorbidity Survey replication. *Archives of General Psychiatry* 62:617–27.

Kessler, R. C., O. Demler, R. G. Frank, et al. 2005. Prevalence and treatment of mental disorders, 1990 to 2003. *New England Journal of Medicine* 352(24):2515–23.

Kessler, R. C., K. A. McGonagle, S. Zhao, et al. 1994. Lifetime and twelve-month prevalence of DSM-III-R psychiatric disorders in the United States: Results from the National Comorbidity Survey. *Archives of General Psychiatry* 51(1):8–19.

Kessler, R. C., C. B. Nelson, K. A. McGonagle, et al. 1996. Comorbidity of DSM-III-R major depressive disorder in the general population: Results from the US National Comorbidity Survey. *British Journal of Psychiatry* (Suppl.) (30):17–30.

Klein, D. F. 1964. Delineation of two drug-responsive anxiety syndromes. *Psychopharmacology* 5:397–408.

Klerman, G. L. 1977. Better but not well: Social and ethical issues in the deinstitutionalization of the mentally ill. *Schizophrenia Bulletin* 3(4):617–31.

Klerman, G. L., P. W. Lavori, J. Rice, et al. 1985. Birth-cohort trends in rates of major depressive disorder among relatives of patients with affective disorder. *Archives of General Psychiatry* 42(7):689–93.

Klerman, G. L., A. Dimascio, M. Weissman, et al. 1974. Treatment of depression by drugs and psychotherapy. *American Journal of Psychiatry* 131:186–91.

Koran, L. M. 1979. Psychiatric manpower ratios. *Archives of General Psychiatry* 36:1409–15.

Kramer, M. 1977. *Psychiatric Services and the Changing Institutional Scene, 1950–1985.* DHEW Publication (ADM) 77–483. Rockville, Md.: Alcohol, Drug Abuse and Mental Health Administration.

———. 1978. Population changes and schizophrenia, 1920–1985. In *The Nature of Schizophrenia,* ed L. C. Wynne. New York: Wiley.

———. 1983. The increasing prevalence of mental disorder: A pandemic threat. *Psychiatric Quarterly* 55:115–43.

Kramer, M., C. A. Taube, and R. W. Redick. 1973. Patterns of use of psychiatric facilities by the aging: Past, present, and future. In *The Psychology of Adult Development and Aging,* ed. C. Eisdorfer and P. M. Lawton. Washington, D.C.: American Psychological Association, 428–528.

Kratochvil, C. J., J. H. Heiligenstein, R. Dittmann, et al. 2002. Atomoxetine and methylphenidate treatment in children with ADHD: A prospective, randomized, open-label trial. *Journal of the American Academy of Child and Adolescent Psychiatry* 41(7): 776–84.

Kulka, R. A., J. Veroff, and E. Douvan. 1979. Social class and the use of professional help for personal problems, 1957 and 1976. *Journal of Health and Social Behavior* 20(1):2–17.

Lave, J. R., and H. H. Goldman. 1990. Medicare financing for mental health care. *Health Affairs* 9(1):19–30.

Le Pen, C., V. Ravily, J. N. Beuzen, and F. Meurgey. 1994. The cost of treatment dropout in depression: A cost benefit analysis of fluoxetine versus tricyclics. *Journal of Affective Disorders* 31(1):1–18.

Lehman, A. F. 1983. The well-being of chronic mental patients. *Archives of General Psychiatry* 40(4):369–73.

Lehman, A. F. 1999. Quality of care in mental health: The case of schizophrenia. *Health Affairs* 18(5):52–65.

Lehman, A. F., N. C. Ward, and L. S. Linn. 1982. Chronic mental patients: The quality of life issue. *American Journal of Psychiatry* 139(10):1271–76.

Lehman, A. F., S. Possidente, and F. Hawker. 1986. The quality of life of chronic patients in a state hospital and in community residences. *Hospital and Community Psychiatry* 37(9):901–7.

Lehman, A. F., and D. M. Steinwachs. 1998. Translating research into practice: The schizophrenia Patient Outcomes Research Team (PORT) treatment recommendations. *Schizophrenia Bulletin* 24(1):1–10.

Leighton, P. C., J. S. Harding, D. S. Macklin, et al. 1963. *Stirling County Study of Psychiatric Disorder and Socio-cultural Environment,* vol. 3. New York: Glencoe Free Press.

Leonard, D. E. 1993. The comparative pharmacology of new antidepressants. *Journal of Clinical Psychology* 54:3–15.

Leonard, H. L., S. E. Swedo, J. L. Rapoport, et al. 1989. Treatment of childhood obsessive-compulsive disorder with Clomipramine and Desipramine: A double-blind crossover comparison. *Archives of General Psychiatry* 46:1088–92.

Leucht, S., K. Wahlbeck, J. Hamann, and W. Kissling. 2003. New generation antipsychotics versus low-potency conventional antipsychotics: A systematic review and meta-analysis. *Lancet* 361(9369):1581–89.

Levine, D. S., and D. R. Levine. 1975. *The Cost of Mental Illness, 1971.* Contract Report to NIMH ADM-42-74-82(OP).

Levitt, E. 1963. Psychotherapy with children: A further evaluation. *Behavioral Research and Therapy* 1:45–51.

Lieberman, J. A., G. Tollefson, M. Tohen, and HGDH Study Group. 2003. Comparative efficacy and safety of atypical and conventional antipsychotic drugs in first-episode psychosis: A randomized, double-blind trial of Olanzapine versus Haloperidol. *American Journal of Psychiatry* 160(8):1396–404.

Lindsay, F. H. 1982. *Science and Engineering Degrees, 1950–1980: A Source Book*. NSF 82-307. Arlington, Va.: National Science Foundation.

Ling, D., A. Busch, and R. G. Frank. 2004. Treatment price indexes for bipolar disorder. Working paper, Harvard University.

Ling, D., R. G. Frank, and E. R. Berndt. 2002. Behavioral health carve-out implementation and diffusion of new psychotropic medications in the Medicaid population. Unpublished manuscript, Harvard University.

Link, B. G., J. C. Phelan, M. Bresnahan, et al. 1999. Public conceptions of mental illness: Labels, causes, dangerousness, and social distance. *American Journal of Public Health* 89(9):1328–33.

Linn, M. W., E. M. Caffey Jr., C. J. Klett, and G. Hogarty. 1977. Hospital vs. community (foster) care for psychiatric patients. *Archives of General Psychiatry* 34(1):78–83.

Liptzin, B. 1979. The psychiatrist shortage. *Archives of General Psychiatry* 36:1416–19.

Long, S., T. Coughlin, and S. J. Kendall. 2002. Access to care among disabled adults on Medicaid. *Health Care Financing Review* 23(4):159–73.

Lopez-Ibor, J. J., and E. Fernandez-Cordoba. 1967. La monoclorimipramina en enfermos resistentes a otros tratamientos: Actas Luso-Espan. *Neurol Psiquiatria* 26:119–47.

Loprest, P. J., and S. R. Zedlewski. 1999. Current and former welfare recipients: How do they differ? In *Assessing the New Federalism. An Urban Institute Program to Assess Changing Social Policies*. Washington, D.C.: Urban Institute.

Luborsky, L., B. Singer, and L. Loborsky. 1975. Comparative studies of psychotherapies: Is it true that "everywon has one and all must have prizes"? *Archives of General Psychiatry* 32(8):33–39.

Lutterman, T. C. 2002. Sixteen state mental health performance indicators. National Association of State Mental Health Program Directors Research Institute, http://nri.rdmc.org/SDICC/SDICC_DIGMeeting.cfm.

Lutterman, T. C., and M. Hogan. 2001. State mental health agency controlled expenditures and revenues for mental health services, 1981 to 1997. In U.S. Dept. of Health and Human Services, Center for Mental Health Services, *Mental Health, United States, 2000*, ed. R. W. Manderscheid and M. J. Henderson. Rockville, Md.: Substance Abuse and Mental Health Services Administration, Center for Mental Health Services, 218–30.

Manderscheid, R. W., J. E. Atay, M. del Hernandez-Cartagena, et al. 2001. Highlights of organized mental health services in 1998 in major national and state trends. In U.S. Dept. of Health and Human Services, Center for Mental Health Services, *Mental Health, United States, 2000*, ed. R. W. Manderscheid and M. J. Henderson. Rockville, Md.: Substance Abuse and Mental Health Services Administration, Center for Mental Health Services, www.mentalhealth.org/publications/allpubs/SMA01-3537/chapter14asp (February 2006).

Manning, W. E., C. F. Liu, T. Stoner, et al. 1999. Outcomes for Medicaid beneficiaries with schizophrenia under a pre-paid mental health carve-out. *Journal of Behavioral Health Services and Research* 26(4):442–50.

March, J. S., A. Frances, D. Carpenter, et al. 1997. Treatment of obsessive-compulsive disorder: The Expert Consensus Panel for obsessive-compulsive disorder. *Journal of Clinical Psychiatry* 58 (Suppl. 4):2–72.

Mark, T. R., R. Coffey, R. Vandivort-Warren, et al. 2005. U.S. spending for mental health and substance abuse treatment, 1991–2001. *Health Affairs* (Web exclusive) W5:133–42.

Marks, I. M. 1981. *Cure and Care of Neuroses: Theory and Practice of Behavioral Psychotherapy.* New York: Wiley.

Marshall, G. N., M. A. Burnam, P. Koegel, et al. 1996. Objective life circumstances and life satisfaction: Results from the course of homelessness study. *Journal of Health and Social Behavior* 37(1):44–58.

Martin, J. K., B. A. Pescosolido, and S. A. Tuch. 2000. Of fear and loathing: The role of "disturbing behavior," labels, and causal attributions in shaping public attitudes toward people with mental illness. *Journal of Health and Social Behavior* 41 (June):208–23.

May, P. R. A. 1968. *Treatment of Schizophrenia: A Comparative Study of Five Treatment Methods.* New York: Science Health.

McAlpine, D. D., and D. Mechanic. 2000. Utilization of speciality mental health care among persons with severe mental illness: The roles of demographics, need, insurance and risk. *Health Services Research* 35(2):277–92.

McGlynn, E. A., S. M. Asch, J. Adams, et al. 2003. The quality of health care delivered to adults in the United States. *New England Journal of Medicine* 348, part 26:2635–45.

McGuire, T. G. 1981. *Financing Psychotherapy: Costs Effects and Public Policy.* Cambridge, Mass.: Ballentine Books.

McGuire, T. G., and J. Montgomery. 1982. Mandated mental health benefits in private health insurance policies. *Journal of Health Politics, Policy and Law* 7(2):380–406.

McSween, J. L. 2002. The role of group interest, identity, and stigma in determining mental health policy preferences. *Journal of Health Politics, Policy and Law* 27(5):773–800.

Mechanic, D. 1969. *Mental Health and Social Policy.* Englewood Cliffs, N.J.: Prentice-Hall.

———. 1989. Toward the year 2000 in U.S. mental health policy making and administration. In *Handbook of Mental Health Policy in the United States*, ed. D. A. Rochefort. Westport, Conn.: Greenwood Press, 477–503.

———. 2003. Is the prevalence of mental disorders a good measure of the need for services? *Health Affairs* 22(5):8–20.

Mechanic, D., and S. Bilder. 2004. Treatment of people with mental illness: A decade-long perspective. *Health Affairs* 23(4):84–95.

Mechanic, D., S. Bilder, and D. D. McAlpine. 2002. Employing persons with serious mental illness. *Health Affairs* 21(5):242–53.

Min DeParle, N. 2000. Celebrating thirty-five years of Medicare and Medicaid. *Health Care Financing Review* 22(1): 1–7.

Minkoff, K. 1978. A map of the chronic mental patient. In *Task Force Report of the American Psychiatric Association Ad Hoc Committee on the Chronic Mental Patient*, by American Psychiatric Association. Washington, D.C.: American Psychiatric Association, 11–37.

Molitch, L., and J. P. Eccles. 1937. Effect of benzedrine sulfate on the intelligence scores of children. *American Journal of Psychiatry* 94:587–90.

Monahan, J., M. Swartz, and R. J. Bonnie. 2003. Mandated treatment in the community for people with mental disorders. *Health Affairs* 22(5):28–38.

Montgomery, S. A., J. Henry, G. MacDonald, et al. 1994. Selective serotonin reuptake inhibitors: A meta-analysis of discontinuation rates. *Internal Clinical Pharmacology* 9:47–53.

Morris, J. B., and A. T. Beck. 1974. The efficacy of antidepressant drugs: A review of research (1958–1972). *Archives of General Psychiatry* 30(5):667–74.

Murphy, J. M., A. M. Sobol, R. K. Neff, et al. 1984. Stability of prevalence: Depression and anxiety disorders. *Archives of General Psychiatry* 41:990–97.

Narrow, W. E., D. S. Rae, L. N. Robins, and D. A. Regier. 2002. Revised prevalence estimates of mental disorders in the United States: Using a clinical significance criterion to reconcile two surveys' estimates. *Archives of General Psychiatry* 59:115–23.

National Center for Health Services Research. 1977. *National Medical Care Expenditure Survey.* 2nd ICPSR release. Hyattsville, Md.: U.S. National Center for Health Services Research.

National Center for Health Statistic. *National Ambulatory Medical Care Survey.* Public-use data file and documentation, ftp://ftp.cdc.gov/pub/Health_Statistics/NCHS/Datasets/ NAMCS/.

———. *National Hospital Discharge Survey.* Public-use data file and documentation, ftp:// ftp.cdc.gov/pub/Health_Statistics/NCHS/Datasets/NHDS/.

National Science Foundation, Division of Science Resources Statistics. 2004. *Science and Engineering Degrees, 1966–2001.* NSF 04-311. Arlington, Va.: National Science Foundation.

Newhouse, J. P., and the Insurance Experiment Group. 1993. *Free for All? Lessons from the RAND Health Insurance Experiment.* Cambridge: Harvard University Press.

Newman, S. J., J. D. Reschovsky, K. Kaneda, and A. M. Hendrick. 1994. The effects of independent living on persons with chronic mental illness: An assessment of the Section 8 certificate program. *Milbank Quarterly* 72(1):171–98.

New York Times. 1955. High cost is cited in mental illness. March 26.

NIH Consensus Development Panel on Depression in Late Life. 1992. Diagnosis and treatment of depression in late life. *Journal of the American Medical Association* 268:1018–24.

NIH Consensus Statement. 1998. Diagnosis and treatment of attention deficit hyperactivity disorder. 16(2):1–37.

Nordhaus, W. D. 2003. The health of nations: The contribution of improved health to living standards. In *Measuring the Gains from Medical Research: An Economic Approach,* ed. K. M. Murphy and R. H. Topel. Chicago: University of Chicago Press, 9–40.

O'Flaherty, B. 1996. *Making Room: The Economics of Homelessness.* Cambridge: Harvard University Press.

Olfson, M., C. S. Marcus, B. Druss, et al. 2002. National trends in the outpatient treatment of depression. *Journal of the American Medical Association* 287(2):203–9.

Pardes, H. 1979. Future needs for psychiatrists and other mental health personnel. *Archives of General Psychiatry* 36:1401–8.

Parloff, M. B. 1984. Cost considerations in psychotherapy. In *Cost Considerations in Mental Health Treatment: Settings, Modalities and Providers,* ed. Z. Taintor, P. Widem, and S. A. Barrett. DHHS Publication (ADM) 84-1295. Washington, D.C.: U.S. Government Printing Office.

Parrott, S., and S. Dean. 2002. Aligning policies and procedures in benefit programs.

Paper prepared for the Center for Budget and Policy Priorities, Washington D.C.

Pasamanick, B. 1962. A survey of mental disease in an urban population: An approach to total prevalence by age. *Mental Hygiene* 46:567–72.

Pasamanick, B., D. W. Roberts, D. W. Lemkau, and D. B. Krueger. 1959. A survey of mental disease in an urban population: Prevalence by race and income. In *Epidemiology of Mental Disorder*, ed. B. Pasamainick. Washington, D.C.: American Association for the Advancement of Society.

Peretti, S., R. Judge, and I. Hindmarch. 2000. Safety and tolerability considerations: Tricyclic antidepressants versus selective serotonin reuptake inhibitors. *Acta Psychiatrica Scandinavica* (Suppl.) 403:17–25.

Pescosolido, B. A., J. Monahan, B. G. Link, et al. 1999. The public's view of the competence, dangerousness, and need for legal coercion of persons with mental health problems. *American Journal of Public Health* 89(9):1339–45.

Phelan, J. C., B. G. Link, A. Stueve, and B. A. Pescosolido. 2000. Public conceptions of mental illness in 1950 and 1996: What is mental illness and is it to be feared? *Journal of Health and Social Behavior* 41 (June):188–207.

Phelps, C. E. 2000. Information diffusion and best practice adoption. In *Handbook of Health Economics*, vol. 1A, ed. A. J. Culyer and J. P. Newhouse. New York: Elsevier, 224–64.

Phillips, C., L. Lux, J. Wildfire, et al. 1995. *Report on the Effects of Regulation on Quality of Care: Analysis of the Effect of Regulation on the Quality of Care in Board and Care Homes.* Washington, D.C.: U.S. Department of Health and Human Services.

Pigott, T. A., and S. M. Seay. 1999. A review of the efficacy of selective serotonin reuptake inhibitors in obsessive-compulsive disorder. *Journal of Clinical Psychiatry* 60(2):101–6.

Pincus, H. A. 2003. Emerging models of depression care: Multi-level strategies. *International Journal of Methods in Psychiatric Research* 12(1):54–63.

Pollack, E. S., and C. A. Taube. 1973. Trends and projections in state hospital use. Paper presented at a symposium on the future role of the state hospital, State University of New York at Buffalo, Division of Community Psychiatry.

Prusoff, B. A., K. R. Merikangas, and M. M. Weissman. 1988. Lifetime prevalence and age of onset of psychiatric disorders: Recall four years later. *Journal of Psychiatric Research* 22:107–17.

Quigley, J. M. 1999. *A Decent Home: Housing Policy in Perspective.* Berkeley: University of California Press.

Radomsky, A. S., and M. W. Otto. 2001. Cognitive-behavioral therapy for social anxiety disorder. *Psychiatric Clinics of North America* 24(4):805–15.

Redlich, F., and S. R. Kellert. 1978. Trends in American mental health. *American Journal of Psychiatry* 135(1):22–28.

Reed, L. S. 1975. *Coverage and Utilization of Care for Mental Health Conditions under Health Insurance, Various Studies, 1973–1974.* Washington, D.C.: American Psychiatric Association.

Regier, D. A., M. E. Farmer, D. S. Rae, et al. 1993. One-month prevalence of mental disorders in the United States and sociodemographic characteristics: The Epidemiologic Catchment Area study. *Acta Psychiatrica Scandinavica* 88(1):35–47.

Regier, D. A., C. T. Kaelber, D. S. Rae, et al. 1998. Limitations of diagnostic criteria and assessment instruments for mental disorders. *Archives of General Psychiatry* 55(2):109–15.

Regier, D. A., and W. E. Narrow. 2002. Defining clinically significant psychopathology with epidemiologic data. In *Defining Psychopathology in the Twenty-first Century: DSM-V and Beyond*, ed. J. E. Helzer and J. J. Judziak. Arlington, Va.: American Psychiatric Publishing, 19–30.

Regier, D. A., W. E. Narrow, M. B. First, and T. Marshall. 2002. The APA classification of mental disorders: Future perspectives. *Psychopathology* 35(2–3):166–70.

Reinehr, R. C. 1975. *The Machine That Oils Itself: A Critical Look at the Mental Health Establishment.* Chicago: Nelson-Hall.

Riggs, J. E., R. L. McGraw, and R. W. Keefover. 1996. Suicide in the United States, 1951–1988: Constant age-period-cohort rates in 40- to 44-year old men. *Comprehensive Psychiatry* 37(3):222–25.

Robins, E., and S. B. Guze. 1970. Establishment of diagnostic validity in psychiatric illness: Its application to schizophrenia. *American Journal of Psychiatry* 126(7):983–87.

Robins, L. N., and D. A. Regier. 1991. *Psychiatric Disorders in America: The Epidemiologic Catchment Area Study.* New York: Free Press.

Robison, L. M., D. A. Sclar, T. L. Skaer, and R. S. Galin. 1999. National trends in the prevalence of attention-deficit/hyperactivity disorder and the prescribing of methylphenidate among school-age children, 1990–1995. *Clinical Pediatrics* 38(4):209–17.

Rogers, E. M. 1995. *The Diffusion of Innovations.* New York: Free Press.

Rosenbach, M. L., and C. J. Ammering. 1997. Trends in part B mental health utilization and expenditures, 1987–1992. *HCFA Review* 19(3):19–42.

Rosenbach, M. L., R. C. Hermann, and R. A. Dorwart. 1997. The use of electroconvulsive therapy in the Medicare population between 1987 and 1992. *Psychiatric Services* 48 (12):1537–42.

Rosenberg, C. E. 2002. The tyranny of diagnosis: Specific entities and individual experience. *Milbank Quarterly* 80(2):237–60.

Rosenfield, S. 1992. Factors contributing to the subjective quality of life of the chronic mentally ill. *Journal of Health and Social Behavior* 33(4):299–315.

Rosenheck, R., J. Cramer, W. Xu, et al. 1997. A comparison of clozapine and haloperidol in hospitalized patients with refractory schizophrenia. Department of Veterans Affairs Cooperative Study Group on Clozapine in Refractory Schizophrenia. *New England Journal of Medicine* 337(12):851–52.

Rosenstein, M. J. 1990. Characteristics of persons using specialty inpatient, outpatient and partial care programs in 1986. In U.S. Department of Health and Human Services, Center for Mental Health Services, *Mental Health, United States, 1990*, ed. R. W. Manderscheid and M. A. Sonnenschein. Rockville, Md.: Substance Abuse and Mental Health Services Administration, Center for Mental Health Services, 139–72.

Rosenthal, M. B., E. R. Berndt, J. M Donohue, et al. 2002. Promotion of prescription drugs to consumers. *New England Journal of Medicine* 346(7):498–505.

Rubin, J. 1978. *Economics, Mental Health and the Law.* Lexington, Mass.: Lexington Books

———. 1980. Judicial standards and the financing of mental health services. *Inquiry* 17(2):165–71.

Rupp, K., and S. H. Bell. 2003. *Paying for Results in Vocational Rehabilitation: Will Provider Incentives Work for Ticket to Work?* Washington, D.C.: Urban Institute Press.

Rush, A. J., A. T. Beck, M. Kovacs, and S. Hollon. 1977. Comparative efficacy of cognitive therapy and pharmacotherapy in the treatment of depressed outpatients. *Cognitive Therapy and Research* (Historical Archive) 1(1):17–37.

Saccar, C. L. 1978. Drug therapy in the treatment of minimal brain dysfunction. *American Journal of Hospital Pharmacy* 35(5):544–52.

Salkever, D. S. 2000. Activity status and perceived productivity for adults with developmental disabilities. *Journal of Rehabilitation* 66(3):4–13.

———. 2003. Tickets without takers? Potential barriers to the supply of rehabilitation services to beneficiaries with mental disorders. In *Paying for Results in Vocational Rehabilitation*, ed. K. Rupp and S. Bell. Washington, D.C.: Urban Institute Press.

Salzer, M. S., J. Rappaport, and L. Segre. 2001. Mental health professionals' support of self-help groups. *Journal of Community and Applied Social Psychology* 11(1):1–10.

Schou, M. 1954. The treatment of manic psychoses by the administration of lithium salts. *Journal of Neurology, Neurosurgery, and Psychiatry* 17:250–60.

Schutt, R., S. Goldfinger, and W. E. Penk. 1997. Satisfaction with residence and with life: When homeless mentally ill persons are housed. *Evaluation and Program Planning* 20(2):185–94.

Schwab, J. J., and G. J. Warheit. 1972. Evaluating southern mental health needs and services: A preliminary report. *Journal of the Florida Medical Association* 59(1):17–20.

Segal, S. P., and P. Kotler. 1989. Community residential care. In *Handbook of Mental Health Policy in the United States*, ed. D. A. Rochefort. Westport, Conn.: Greenwood Press.

Sempos, C. T., J. I. Cleeman, M. D. Carroll, et al. 1993. Prevalence of high blood cholesterol among U.S. adults: An update based on guidelines from the second report of the National Cholesterol Education Program Adult Treatment Panel. *Journal of the American Medical Association* 269(23):3009–14.

Shadish, W. R., A. J. Lurigo, and D. A. Lewis. 1989. After deinstitutionalization: The present and future of mental health long term care policy. *Journal of Social Issues* 45(3):1–15.

Shaffer, D., P. Fisher, M. K. Dulcan, et al. 1996. The NIMH Diagnostic Interview Schedule for Children version 2.3 (DISC-2.3): Description, acceptability, prevalence rates, and performance in the MECA Study. Methods for the Epidemiology of Child and Adolescent Mental Disorders Study. *Journal of the American Academy of Child and Adolescent Psychiatry* 35:865–77.

Sharfstein, S. S. 2000. Whatever happened to community mental health? *Psychiatric Services* 51(5):616–20.

Shen, Y. 1999. A history of antipsychotic drug development. *Comprehensive Psychiatry* 40(6):407–14.

Shore, J. H., J. D. Kinzie, J. L. Hampson, and E. M. Pattison. 1973. Psychiatric epidemiology of an Indian village. *Psychiatry* 36(1):70–81.

Shore, M. F., and M. D. Cohen. 1990. The Robert Wood Johnson Foundation Program on Chronic Mental Illness: An overview. *Hospital and Community Psychiatry* 41(11):1212–16.

Shorter, E. 1997. *A History of Psychiatry: From the Year of the Asylum to the Age of Prozac.* New York: Wiley.

Signorielli, N. 1989. The stigma of mental illness on television. *Journal of Broadcasting and Electronic Media* 33(3):325–31.

Simon, G. E., and M. VonKorff. 1992. Reevaluation of secular trends in depression rates. *American Journal of Epidemiology* 135(12):1411–22.

Sinaiko, R. J., and T. G. McGuire. 2005. Patient inducement, provider priorities and resource allocation in public mental health systems. Working paper, Harvard University.

Sirey, J. A., M. L. Bruce, G. Alexopoulos, et al. 2001. Perceived stigma and patient-rated severity of illness as predictors of antidepressant drug adherence. *Psychiatric Services* 52(12):1615–20.

Sledge, W. H., J. Tebes, N. Wolff, and T. W. Helminiak. 1996. Day hospital/crisis respite care versus inpatient care, part II: Service utilization and costs. *American Journal of Psychiatry* 153:1074–83.

Somers, H. M., and A. R. Somers. 1961. *Doctors, Patients and Health Insurance.* Washington, D.C.: Brookings Institution Press.

Song, F., N. Freemantle, T. A. Sheldon, et al. 1993. Selective serotonin reuptake inhibitors: Meta-analysis of efficacy and acceptability. *BMJ* 306(6879):683–87.

Spencer, T., J. Biederman, and T. Wilens. 1994. Tricyclic antidepressant treatment of children with ADHD and tic disorders. *Journal of American Academy of Child and Adolescent Psychiatry* 33(8):1203–4.

Spitzer, R. L., J. Endicott, and E. Robins. 1975. *Research Diagnostic Criteria.* New York: Biometrics Research Division, New York State Psychiatric Institute.

Srole, L. 1962. *Mental Health in the Metropolis: The Midtown Manhattan Study.* New York: McGraw-Hill.

Srole, L., T. S. Lagner, S. T. Michael, et al. 1978. *Mental Health in the Metropolis: The Midtown Manhattan Study.* Rev. ed. New York: New York University Press.

Stapleton, D., K. Coleman, K. Dietrich, and G. Livermore. 1998. Empirical analyses of DI and SSI application and award growth. In *Growth in Disability Benefits,* ed. K. Rupp and D. Stapleton. Kalamazoo, Mich.: W. E. Upjohn Institute for Employment Research.

Star, S. A. 1952. *What the Public Thinks about Mental Health and Mental Illness.* Chicago: National Opinion Research Center.

———. 1955. The public's ideas about mental illness. Paper presented at the annual meeting of the National Association for Mental Health, Indianapolis, November 5.

Starr, P. 1982. *The Social Transformation of American Medicine.* New York: Basic Books.

Stroup, T. S., J. P. McEvoy, M. S. Swartz, et al. 2003. The National Institute of Mental Health Clinical Antipsychotic Trials of Intervention Effectiveness (CATIE) project: Schizophrenia trial design and protocol development. *Schizophrenia Bulletin* 29(1):15–31.

Sturm, R. 1999. Tracking changes in behavioral health services: How have carve-outs changed care? *Journal of Behavioral Health Services and Research* 26(4):360–71.

Sturm, R., and R. Klap. 1999. Use of psychiatrists, psychologists, and master's-level therapists in managed behavioral health care carve-out plans. *Psychiatric Services* 50(4):504–8.

Sturm, R., and K. B. Wells. 2000. Health insurance may be improving but not for individuals with mental illness. *Health Services* 35(1)2:253–62.

Swanson, J., M. Lerner, and L. Williams. 1995. More frequent diagnosis of attention deficit-hyperactivity disorder. *New England Journal of Medicine* 333:944.

Syzmanski, H. V., H. C. Schulberg, V. Salter, et al. 1982. Estimating the local prevalence of persons needing community support programs. *Hospital and Community Psychiatry* 33:370–73.

Szasz, T. S. 1976. *Schizophrenia: The Sacred Symbol of Psychiatry.* New York: Basic Books.
———. 1987. *Insanity: The Idea and Its Consequences.* New York: Wiley.
Talbott, J. A., ed. 1978. *The Chronic Mental Patient: Problems, Solutions, and Recommendations for Public Policy.* Washington, D.C.: American Psychiatric Association.
Talbott, J. A., and S. S. Sharfstein. 1986. A proposal for future funding of chronic and episodic mental illness. *Hospital and Community Psychiatry* 37(11):1126–30.
Teplin, L. A. 1990. The prevalence of severe mental disorder among male urban jail detainees: Comparison with the Epidemiologic Catchment Area program. *American Journal of Public Health* 80:663–69.
Thomas, L. 1974. *The Lives of a Cell.* New York. Viking Press.
Todorov, C., M. H. Freeston, and F. Borgeat. 2000. On the pharmacotherapy of obsessive-compulsive disorder: Is a consensus possible? *Canadian Journal of Psychiatry* 45:257–62.
Trindade, E., D. Menon, L. A. Topfer, and C. Coloma. 1998. Adverse effects associated with selective serotonin reuptake inhibitors and tricyclic antidepressants: A meta-analysis. *Canadian Medical Association Journal* 159(10):1245–52.
Trussell, R. E., J. Elinson, and M. L. Levin. 1956. Comparisons of various methods of estimating the prevalence of chronic disease in a community: The Hunterdon County study. *American Journal of Public Health* 46: 173–82.
U.S. Army Medical Service. 1966. *Neuropsychiatry in World War II.* Washington, D.C.: Office of the Surgeon General, Department of the Army.
U.S. Bureau of the Census. 1990. Persons in group quarters: Census of the population, 1990. www.census.gov/population/www/censusdata/grpqtr.html.
———. 2000. Census 2000 summary file 1, matrix PCT17. QT-P12. Group quarters population by sex, age, and type of group quarters. http://factfinder.census.gov.
U.S. Congress. 1981. Omnibus Reconciliation Act of 1981.
U.S. Department of Agriculture. 2001. Characteristics of food stamp households: Fiscal year 2001 (advance report). www.fns.usda.gov/oane/MENU/Published/FSP/FILES/Participation/2001AdvSum.htm.
U.S. Department of Health, Education and Welfare. 1980. *Mental Health and the Elderly.* Publication 80-20960. Washington, D.C.: U.S. General Accounting Office.
U.S. Department of Health and Human Services. 1980. *Toward a National Plan for the Chronically Mentally Ill: Report to the Secretary.* Washington, D.C.: U.S. DHHS.
———. *National Medical Expenditure Survey, 1987.* 1992. Rockville, Md.: Agency for Health Care Policy and Research.
———. 1993. *Depression Guidelines Panel: Treatment of Depression.* AHCPR Publication 930551. Rockville, Md.: Agency for Health Care Policy and Research.
———. 1999. *Treatment of Depression: Newer Pharmacotherapies.* Evidence Report/Technology Assessment 7, Publication 99-E014. Rockville, Md.: Agency for Health Care Policy and Research.
U.S. Department of Health and Human Services, Agency for Healthcare Research and Quality. 2005. *Medical Expenditure Panel Survey.* www.meps.ahrq.gov/Puf/PUFLookup.asp.
U.S. Department of Health and Human Services, Center for Mental Health Services. 1985. *Mental Health, United States 1985,* ed. C. A. Taube and S. A. Barrett. Rockville, Md.: Alcohol, Drug Abuse and Mental Health Administration.

———. 1994. *Mental Health, United States 1994*. Rockville, Md.: Substance Abuse and Mental Health Services Administration, Center for Mental Health Services.

———. 1999. *Mental Health: A Report of the Surgeon General*. Rockville, Md.: Substance Abuse and Mental Health Services Administration, Center for Mental Health Services.

———. 2001a. *Mental Health: Culture, Race, and Ethnicity. A Report of the Surgeon General*. Rockville, Md.: Substance Abuse and Mental Health Services Administration, Center for Mental Health Services.

———. 2001b. *Mental Health, United States, 2000*, ed. R. W. Manderscheid and M. J. Henderson. Rockville, Md.: Substance Abuse and Mental Health Services Administration, Center for Mental Health Services.

———. 2003. *Health, U.S.* Washington, D.C.: U.S. Department of Health and Human Services.

———. 2004. *Mental Health, United States, 2002*, ed. R. W. Manderscheid and M. J. Henderson. DHHS Publication (SMA) 3938. Rockville, Md.: Substance Abuse and Mental Health Services Administration, Center for Mental Health Services.

U.S. Department of Housing and Urban Development. 1990. Report of Congress on SROs for the homeless Section 8 moderate rehabilitation program.

———. 1993. Consolidated annual report to Congress on fair housing programs.

———. 1995. Lower income housing assistance program (Section 8) interim findings of evaluation research.

———. 2000. Section 8 tenant-based housing assistance: A look back after thirty years. www.huduser.org/publications/pdf/look.pdf.

U.S. Food and Drug Administration. Orange Book. www.fda.gov/cder/ob/default.htm (most recent update November 2005).

U.S. General Accounting Office. 1977. *Returning the Mentally Disabled to the Community: Government Needs to Do More*. Washington, D.C.: U.S. GAO.

———. 1999. *ONDCP Efforts to Manage the National Drug Control Budget*. Washington, D.C.: General Accounting Office.

U.S. Health Care Financing Administration. 1992. *Report to Congress: Medicaid and Institutions for Mental Disease*. HCFA Publication 03339. Washington, D.C.: U.S Health Care Financing Administration.

U.S. House of Representatives, Committee on Ways and Means. 2000. *2000 Green Book*. Publication WMCP 106-14. Washington, D.C.: Government Printing Office.

———. 2004. *2004 Green Book*. Publication WMCP 108-6. Washington, D.C.: Government Printing Office.

U.S. President's Commission on Mental Health. 1978a. *Report to the President from the President's Commission on Mental Health*. Washington, D.C.: Government Printing Office.

———. 1978b. *Task Panel Reports*, vol. 2. Washington, D.C.: U.S. Government Printing Office.

U.S. President's New Freedom Commission on Mental Health. 2003. *Achieving the Promise: Transforming Mental Health Care in America. Final Report*. DHHS Publication SMA-03-3832. Rockville, Md.: President's New Freedom Commission on Mental Health.

U.S. Social Security Administration. 2001. *Annual Statistical Supplement to the Social Security Bulletin*. Washington, D.C.: U.S. Government Printing Office.

————. 2004. *Annual Statistical Supplement to the Social Security Bulletin*. Washington, D.C.: U.S. Government Printing Office.

Van Putten, T., and R. P. May. 1978. "Akinetic depression" in schizophrenia. *Archives of General Psychiatry* 35(9):1101–7.

Wahl, O. F. 1996. Schizophrenia in the news. *Psychiatric Rehabilitation Journal* 20(1):51–55.

————. 1999. Mental health consumers' experience of stigma. *Schizophrenia Bulletin* 25(3):467–78.

Wahl O. F., L. Borostovik, and R. Rieppi. 1995. Schizophrenia in popular periodicals. *Community Mental Health Journal* 31(3):239–48.

Wahl, O. F., and A. L. Kaye. 1992. Mental illness topics in popular periodicals. *Community Mental Health Journal* 28(1):21–28.

Wakefield, J. C., and R. L. Spitzer. 2002. Why requiring clinical significance does not solve epidemiology's and DSM's validity problem. In *Defining Psychopathology in the Twenty-first Century: DSM-V and Beyond*, ed. J. E. Helzer and J. J. Hudziak. Arlington, Va.: American Psychiatric Publishing.

Weissman, M. M., and G. Klerman. 1980. Psychiatric nosology and the midtown Manhattan study. *Archives of General Psychiatry* 37:229–30.

Weissman, M. M., J. K. Myers, and P. S. Harding. 1978. Psychiatric disorders in a U.S. urban community, 1975–1976. *American Journal of Psychiatry* 135(4):459–62.

Weissman, M. M., J. K. Myers, and W. D. Thompson. 1981. Depression and its treatment in a US urban community, 1975–1976. *Archives of General Psychiatry* 38(4):417–21.

Wernicke, J. F., and C. J. Kratochvil. 2002. Safety profile of atomoxetine in the treatment of children and adolescents with ADHD. *Journal of Clinical Psychiatry* 63 (Suppl. 12):50–55.

West, J., J. Kohout, G. M. Pion, et al. 2001. Mental health practitioners and trainees. In *Mental Health, United States, 2000*, ed. R. W. Manderscheid and M. J. Henderson. Rockville, Md.: Substance Abuse and Mental Health Services Administration, Center for Mental Health Services, 279–315.

Wickramaratne, P. J., M. M. Weissman, P. J. Leaf, and T. R. Holford. 1989. Age, period and cohort effects on the risk of major depression: Results from five United States communities. *Journal of Clinical Epidemiology* 42(4):333–43.

Williams, L. D. 1990. Businesses facing rising mental health costs are turning to managed care. *Baltimore Sun*, August 5.

Witkin, M. J., J. Atay, and R. W. Manderscheid. 1996. Trends in state and county mental hospitals in the U.S. from 1970–1992. *Psychiatric Services* 47(10):1079–81.

Wolpe, J. 1958. *Psychotherapy by Reciprocal Inhibition*. Stanford: Stanford University Press.

World Health Organization. 2001. *The World Health Report, 2001—Mental Health: New Understanding, New Hope*. Geneva: World Health Organization (www.who.int/whr/).

Yellin, E. H., and M. G. Cisternas. 1996. Employment patterns among persons with and without mental conditions. In *Mental Disorder, Work Disability, and the Law*, ed. R. J. Bonnie and J. Monahan. Chicago: University of Chicago Press.

Zito, J., D. Safer, S. dosReis, et al. 2000. Trends in the prescribing of psychotropic medications to preschoolers. *Journal of the American Medical Association* 283:1025–30.

Richard G. Frank, PhD, is the Margaret T. Morris Professor of Health Economics in the Department of Health Care Policy at Harvard Medical School. He is also a research associate with the National Bureau of Economic Research. Dr. Frank is engaged in research in three general areas: the economics of mental health care, the economics of the pharmaceutical industry, and the organization and financing of physician group practices. He serves on the Congressional Citizens' Working Group on Health Care. He advises several state mental health and substance abuse agencies on issues related to managed care and financing of care. In 1997 Dr. Frank was elected to the Institute of Medicine. He has been awarded the Georgescu-Roegen prize from the Southern Economic Association for work on drug pricing, the Carl A. Taube Award from the American Public Health Association, and the Emily Mumford Medal from Columbia University's Department of Psychiatry. In 2002 Dr. Frank received the John Eisberg Mentorship Award from National Research Service Awards.

Sherry A. Glied is a professor and the chair of the Department of Health Policy and Management of Columbia University's Mailman School of Public Health. She holds a BA in economics from Yale University, an MA in economics from the University of Toronto, and a PhD in economics from Harvard University. In 1992–93 she served as a senior economist for health care and labor market policy on the President's Council of Economic Advisers, under both President Bush and President Clinton. In the latter part of her term she was a participant in President Clinton's Health Care Task Force. Professor Glied's principal areas of research are health policy reform and mental health care policy. Her research has focused on the financing of health care services in the United States. She is an author of many articles and reports on managed care, the design of health insurance expansions, child health and mental health, and women's health. Her book on health care reform, *Chronic Condition*, was published by Harvard University

Press in 1998. In 2004 Professor Glied was chair of the Annual Research Meeting of Academy Health, the professional organization of health services researchers and health policy analysts. She was the 2004 winner of Research!America's Eugene Garfield Economic Impact of Medical and Health Research Award.